# YOGA

The Best 110 Poses for Practice, Guide and Tips for Improving Your Health

Inna Volia

# Contents

# Introduction

Yoga as a science has gained such a widespread popularity with many people embracing it considering the diverse benefits that the practice is associated with. Yoga doesn't only provide a great way of exercising and relaxation, it equally enables people to connect deeply with whom they truly are which then leads to higher levels of consciousness and self-awareness. The practice of yoga is associated with diverse benefits that people get to realize when they are more self-aware. They are able to focus their energies on things that matter most to them and will be able to take actions that are beneficial to their lives.

Taking time to understand yoga is vital if one is to experience the various improvements and benefits that come with practicing yoga. Their practice of yoga entails various practices such as postures, breathing and meditation and all of them when done with understanding lead one to experience union. This book has shared in detail the science of yoga and all that it entails. The book has covered the history of yoga, the various ways in which the practice of yoga can be used to improve one's life and the well being. It's also packed with several yoga poses, the steps to follow for practicing them and the diverse benefits associated with practicing yoga postures.

Take your time to go through the entire book and gain understanding of what yoga is all about. You can also sample out the yoga postures that you can try out depending on your level with the practice. Remember that some postures are suitable for those who are already well versed with yoga practice; trying them out if you're just a beginner may not be quite ideal. It's therefore important that you look out for postures that suit your level so as to avoid unnecessary injuries and pain that may occur due to lack of experience.

Before you start with the postures, it's advisable that you take time and understand what the science entails. There are various types of yoga postures such as the standing postures the sitting yoga postures, the lying down postures and stomach yoga postures, and the lying down on the back yoga postures. Each of the postures addresses different areas of the body as well as the mind, therefore, balancing them is ideal if one is to realize great benefits. Take your time and go through the entire book and for more understanding about yoga and how if well implemented has the potential of improving your life in all areas.

As your level of understanding increases with the practice, you can also progress to the less complex postures and practice them until you're well versed with them. Once you're well versed with the level then you can try out the more advanced and complex yoga postures. Trying out some of this complex postures may require the help of a yoga teacher so precaution should be taken. Engaging in breathing exercises and meditation is key and should be part of the yoga practice. There are yoga postures that are suitable for breathing and for meditation so practicing them when meditating is important.

Thank you for taking your time to invest in this book and I encourage you to read all through; you'll definitely get valuable information as you read.

# Chapter 1

# Understanding Yoga

## What is yoga?

The word yoga when mentioned ignites a few thoughts with some assuming that it means the engaging in certain poses, others relate it to breathing exercises while some see it as a way of meditation. Yoga can, however, be defined as a science that's done with the intention of gaining harmony between the mind and the body. The practice of yoga consists of a set of practices which are spiritual, mental and physical. Practicing yoga involves engaging in spiritual practices or disciplines such as breath control, specific body postures, and meditation. Majority of the people practice yoga mostly for relaxation and for good health, however incorporation all the aspects can be of great help to the body.

Yoga means union or a practice that brings one to an experiential reality where one gets to understand the nature of existence which brings tremendous experience of life. In the day to day life, people often look outside themselves for solutions to issues that they may not be able to understand. The practice of yoga therefore is focused towards enabling one to be in union with their inner self and who they truly are. Real fulfillment comes when someone is able to tap to that power from within them for joy and fulfillment. Looking for joy or happiness from the outside may not provide sustainable feelings of joy. The world that we live in has conditioned people to look for fulfillment from other areas apart from within, a fact that lives many people depressed and burnt out as they lack insight on how to get that which they seek.

The deep longing of man cannot be fulfilled with the superficial outside forces; it's something that one only gets to enjoy when they learn how to connect with their inner self. When you look for fulfillment from external sources then you will always find yourself busy with doing things that enable you to attain the fulfillment but that's what yoga teaches that it's about being in harmony. When your mind and body is in harmony with the universal forces then it puts one in a place where they enjoy higher levels of consciousness and self-awareness. Practicing yoga enables one to be in that place of complete calmness where their feelings and their thoughts seize to be and they are able to enjoy every moment with more clarity and understanding.

It's by being in such a state of calmness that one is capable of accessing the deeper levels of joy and understanding which is quite impossible to attain in any other way. Yoga therefore as an ancient spiritual science helps with stilling the natural turbulence of restlessness and the thoughts that hinder people from knowing who they really are.

Most of the times, people direct their energies and the sense of awareness to external things which are in most of the cases perceived through the physical senses. It, therefore, means that one's capability is limited to the extent to which they can achieve from the senses. Since human beings have to rely on the information received through the physical senses it's important that we learn how to tap deeper and into more subtle levels of awareness so as to be able to solve the complex issues of life. Yoga, therefore, is a process that reverses the general outward flow of energy. The mind then becomes dynamic in the sense that one's perception is no longer dependent on the limited physical senses but is exposed to another dimension of awareness that enables them to experience the truth.

Practicing yoga cultivates that sense of being in unity with the universal forces. The various yoga postures enable one to know of oneness with the universal power which then results in an inflow of self-realization. Yoga is, therefore, a union of the individual consciousness. As much as many people think of yoga as just a set of physical exercises, the exercises are just the superficial aspect of the profound science that aids the unfolding of the infinite potential embedded in the human's mind and soul. The understanding of yoga can, however, be complex as it includes thousands of interpretations and pathways which then lead to expanded consciousness, spiritual awareness and physical fitness.

## History of Yoga

The word yoga originates from the Sanskrit root word Yuj which means to join, to unite or to yoke.  According to the yogic scriptures; practicing yoga results into a union of the individual consciousness with the universal consciousness. It then expresses a perfect harmony between man and nature, the body, and the mind. A person who gets to experience the oneness of existence is considered to be in yoga and is referred to as a yogi. The practice of yoga is said to have begun during the dawn of civilization. However, the origin extends to thousands of years before the discovery of various religions or belief systems. It's preciously begun over 5000 years.

The first yogi also knew as Adiyogi was known as Shiva who shared his knowledge several years ago along the banks of Lake Kantisarovar which is found in the Himalayas. Adiyogi shared his knowledge with the seven sages also known as Saptarishis. The sages then carried the powerful yogic science to various parts of the world such as Asia, Northern Africa, Middle East and South America. The yogic system, however, found full expression in India. Agastya, who was the Saptarishi traveled the entire Indian subcontinent and shared the culture around the yogic way of life. A look at the number of fossil remains that have yogic motives alongside figures performing yoga expresses the spread of yoga in ancient India.

The presence of yoga could be seen in the folk traditions, the Vedic and Upanishadic heritage, the Buddhist and Jain traditions, the Darshanas and more. There was a time when the practice of yoga was limited only to be done by a guru and the spiritual value of yoga was given a lot of importance. A much as yoga was practiced during the pre-Vedic period, Maharshi Patanjali, the greatest sage systemized and codified the practice including its meaning and the related knowledge through yoga sutras which led to conservation of the practice. Historians are not sure of the exact time in which the practice of yoga began however some has attributed it to be between 3300 – 1500 BCE.

## The Eight Fold Path of Yoga

The eight steps of yoga often act as a guideline on how you can live a meaningful and a purposeful life as you practice yoga. The steps serve as a moral prescription or an ethical path that every practitioner should be aware of. They help with directing one towards deeper understanding of yoga and how the practice gets to improve one's life.

### Yama

Deals with the ethical standards as one is expected to cultivate that sense of integrity as they focus on their behavior and conduct as they go through life. It's associated with one acknowledging the golden rule of doing unto others what you expect them to do for you. The five yamas are based on the following qualities: nonviolence, truthfulness, nonstealing, continence and no covetousness.

### Niyama

The second limb as commonly referred to or step is focused on spiritual observances and self-discipline. It entails giving emphasis to spiritual practices such as meditation and other spiritual acts. The five niyamas include; cleanliness, contentment, heat, study of scriptures and surrender to god.

### Asana

This step entails the postures that are practiced in yoga which comprises of the third limb. According to yogic view, the body is considered as the temple of the spirit and how the spirit is cared for is quite important for spiritual growth. Practicing the asanas enables one to develop discipline that spiritual growth requires. One also gets to develop the concentration that's required for meditation.

### Pranayama

It can be translated to breathe control and entails techniques that enables one to gain mastery over breathing and the respiratory process. It also focuses on recognition of the breath, the emotions, and the mind. Pranayama is believed to not only rejuvenate the body but to also extend life. It's advisable that one integrates it into their daily yoga practice.

## Pratyahara

It means sensory transcendence or withdrawal. It's at this stage that one makes the conscious effort to draw their awareness away from the outside world and any other outside stimuli. The withdrawals allow one to objectively observe their life, cravings and other habits that may be detrimental to their health and overall wellbeing.

## Dharana

At this stage, one gets to learn the practice of concentration which often precedes meditation. One gets to learn how to slow the process of thinking as they concentrate on a single mental object. Remember the previous steps such as posture, breath control and the withdrawal of senses helped in building concentration, however, this stage focuses on developing intense concentration where the focus is on a single thing.

## Dhyana

This stage entails contemplation or meditation. It's where one practices a flow of concentration that's uninterrupted. The mind at this stage has been quieted and stillness attained with no thoughts at all. It's important to remember that it takes practice and stamina to get to this stage.

## Samadhi

This is the final stage and is described as the stage of ecstasy where one gets to realize profound connection with the divine and all living things. Such a realization comes with peace that's beyond understanding. Remember that the ultimate stage of yoga is enlightenment which can only be attained through practice and devotion.

# Chapter 2

## Examples of how Yoga Changes and Improves Life

The transformative power of practicing yoga is something that many people have attested to especially those with quality understanding of what the yoga science entails. When practicing yoga, it's important to note that some of the transformations may occur at a subtle and organic level which makes it difficult to point out at what exactly about yoga that led to the transformation being experienced. Embracing the practice of yoga is not just about being flexible and attaining the beautiful postures it also entails exploring the feeling throughout the practice which then enables one to rediscover that sense of wholeness in their life.

Yoga has been proven to change lives in many ways and it's possible to enjoy the benefits if you put this spiritual science into practice. Remember that it's not only about making poses but also monitoring your breathing and reflecting on meditation. Below are some of the ways in which yoga changes and improves life;

**Ideal for all-round fitness**

Health is not just the absence of disease; it's a dynamic way through which life is expressed. Yoga practice enhances the realization of an all-round fitness such as spiritual, mental and physical health and well being. Engaging in yoga postures and meditation helps in improving health, increases mental strength and improves physical strength. It also protects from injury and detoxifies the body alongside other fitness benefits. Engaging in yoga also helps in improving one's intuition which then leads to positive outcomes as one is capable of getting insight regarding things that may not be obvious.

## Weight Loss

There are yoga postures that are known to enhance weight loss. Engaging in regular yoga practice has the potential of influencing weight loss.  Poses like sun salutations help with weight loss if practiced effectively. As much as many yoga practices lead to the burning of fewer calories when compared to the traditional ways of exercising; engaging in yoga practices such as mindfulness and meditation can in a great way impact the overall health and wellbeing of an individual. The benefit of weight loss can be realized by changing the intake and expenditure of energy. Becoming more aware of the foods being consumed and the impact they can have on the body helps in addressing the issue of weight.

Most of the people consume a lot of food when they are under stress and since practicing yoga relieves of tress; it will then be much easier to lose weight. To lose weight through yoga, you have to join a yoga class that challenges you. You have to engage in exercises that cause your heart to beat faster. Engage in something more than relaxation and mindfulness exercises.

## Stress relief and Inner Peace

As much as we enjoy visiting serene spots and peaceful places that are rich in natural beauty, practicing yoga enables one to realize inner peace that can be enjoyed without visiting any outward place. You can have an experience of a holiday every day as you practice yoga and meditation. Yoga also helps in calming a mind filled with stress and anxiety. It fosters inward focus which then causes one to be more aware of their feelings and the daily activities they engage in. Having such a level of self-awareness causes a shift in one's way of thinking, how they treat themselves and their body and the things they spend their energy on.

Once self-awareness is realized; one is able to gain a sense of psychological, emotional and physical realities that get to shift as one gets less influenced by the external forces and more inwardly attuned. The practice of yoga enhances mindfulness which then impacts every aspect of one's being. Practicing yoga also relieves from stress which gets to accumulate daily in the mind and the body. Combining yoga postures with meditation are effective techniques that help with stress relief. The mind is always involved in activities with thoughts that keep rising every time.

Getting the mind to stay in the present moment takes effort and practicing yoga enables the mind to stay in the present moment where one can enjoy being focused and happy.

**Increased Energy and Vitality**

Engaging in yoga practice helps with enhancing one's energetic level and increases vitality. If you find yourself feeling drained by the end of every day or feeling exhausted after a few tasks then spending a few minutes in yoga practice can provide that much-needed energy boost. Yoga practice also enhances flexibility and posture. However, the practice should be part of your daily routine if the desired results are to be realized. Engaging in regular yoga practice helps in stretching and toning the body muscles which then causes them to be strong.

The body posture also gets to improve which then relieves the body of any pain that may arise as a result of poor body posture.

# Chapter 3

## 110 Yoga Poses with Pictures

Practicing yoga poses comes with numerous benefits and may have a great impact on one's overall life and well being. Below are some of the yoga poses that you can consider practicing.

## 1. Bridge Posture

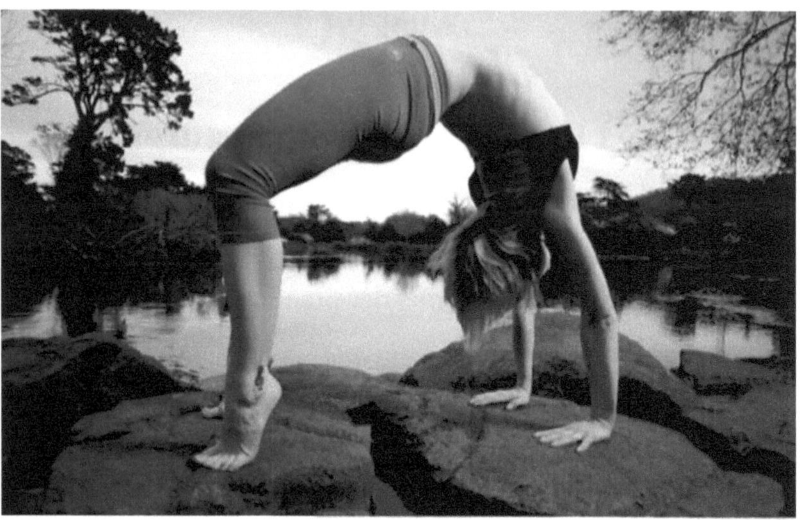

## Steps

- Lie on the ground then lift your upper and lower body as shown in the pose.

- Breathe deeply while in the position for about 30 seconds.

- Relax as you bring down your body as if in a starting position

- You can repeat the cycle for about 5 times.

## Benefits

- Opening the hip joints while also opening the heart and the chest.

- Strengthens the chest and the back while also improving the spinal muscles.

- Reduces stress.

## 2. Easy Pose

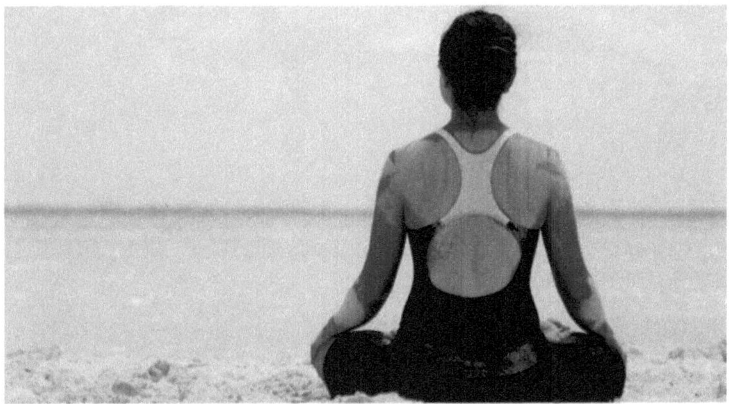

## Steps

- Sit on the floor normally then stretch the legs in front of you

- Cross your legs as you broaden the knees such that your thighs and the legs form a triangle.

- Keep space between your pelvis and feet as your back remains straight and your gaze focused ahead.

- Stay in the position as you take deep long breaths.

## Benefits

- Stretches and lengthens the spine

- The pose helps with opening of the hips and also eases menstrual pains.

- Calms and helps in lowering anxiety levels.

- Enhance peace and serenity

## 3. Triangle Pose

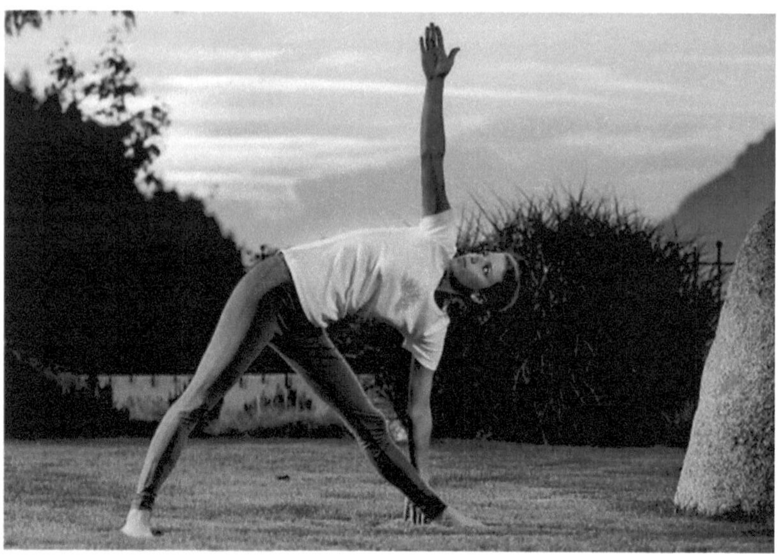

## Steps

- Stand and keep both your feet apart as shown in the pose.

- Turn the right leg to about 90 degrees then breathe in.

- Bend the left side of the body as you exhale and your right hand facing upwards as your left hand touch your left toe.

- Stay with the pose for about 2 minutes then change the other side.

## Benefits

- Improved flexibility of the spine and alignment of the shoulders

- Relief from stiffness around the neck area and back pain.

- Stretches the entire body while also improving blood circulation and stimulated kidney functioning.

## 4. Four limbed staff

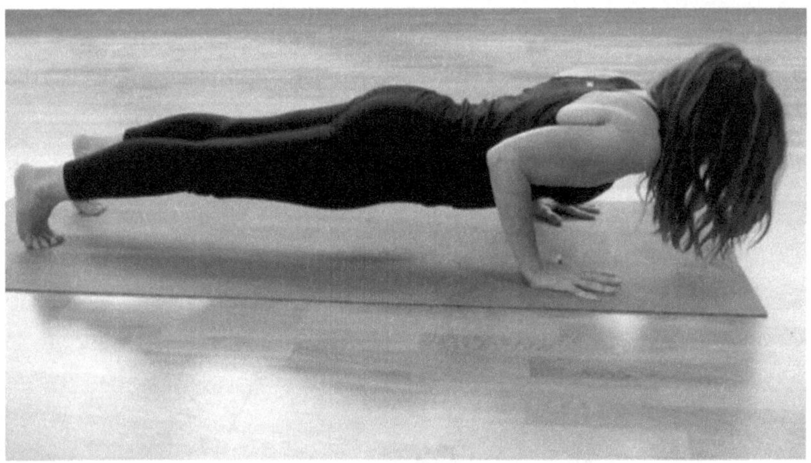

## Steps

- Take standing forward fold then step the feet back into a push-up position.

- Spread your fingers wide apart as you press into your palms with straight arms.

- Tuck your tail bone so that your hips, torso, and legs are in a straight line.

- Press your head forward with your toss tucked as you press the heels back.

- Stay in the position as you breathe and hold four breaths.

## Benefits

- Strengthens the arms, abdomen and the wrists. It can also be used for preparation for more challenging arm balancing poses.

- Lengthens the spine while also strengthening the low back muscles.

## 5.  King dancer pose

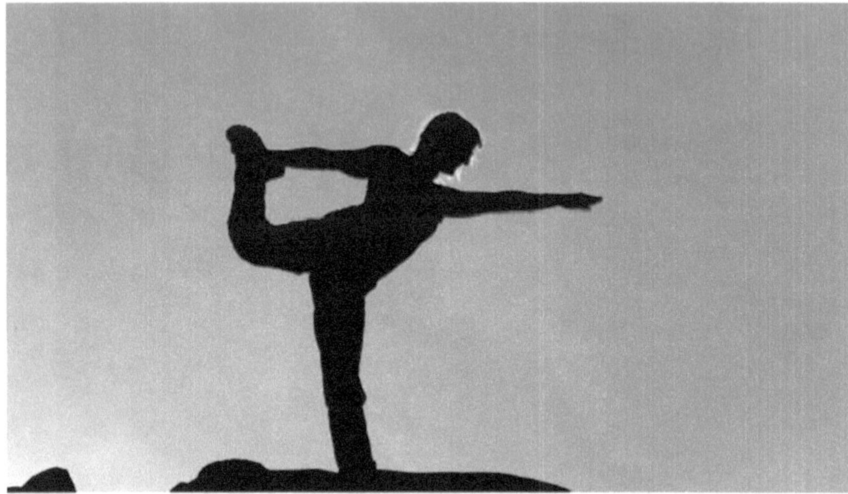

## Steps

- Stand tall with the body weight distributed to the feet.

- Shift your weight to the right foot as you bend the left knee and lift your left feet off the floor.

- Hold the instep of the left foot with the left hand with your thumb resting on the sole of your foot.

- Lift your right arm straight upwards.

- Stay in the position as you take 10 breaths then change to the other foot.

## Benefits

This pose helps with strengthening the legs, while also improving balance and core strength. It also stretches and improves ones focus. It's considered as one of the most graceful

## 6. Warrior pose

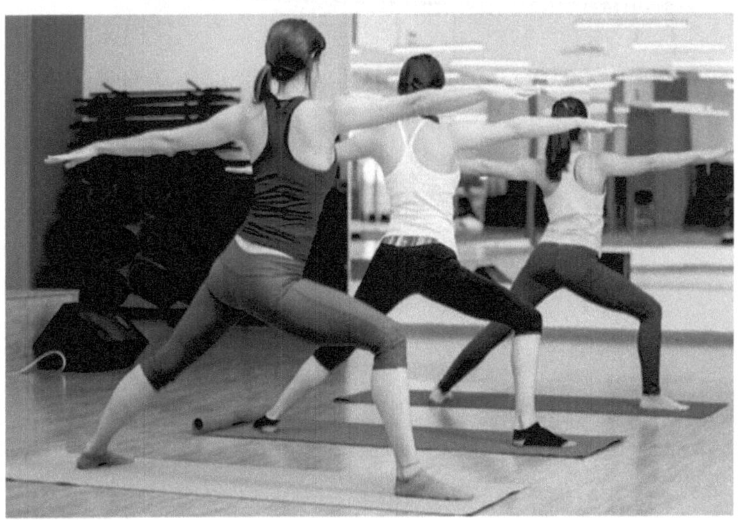

## Steps

- Stand straight with your legs slightly apart.

- Inhale and raise both the hands as you turn your head to the right.

- Exhale as you turn your right foot to about 90 degrees towards the right.

- Bend your knees as demonstrated in the pose as you as you hold for a few minutes.

- Repeat the steps with the left leg as you also turn your head to the left.

## Benefits

- Increases stamina and  flexibility of the whole body

- Strengthens the legs, lower back, the arms and also tones the lower body.

- Strengthens abdominal organs while also improving blood circulation all through the body.

- Relieves stress and pains while also improving concentration.

## 7. Tree Pose

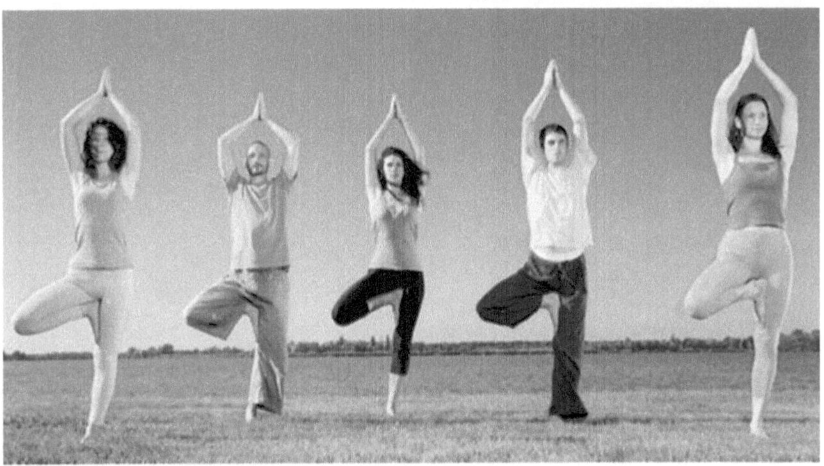

## Steps

- Stand straight with your arms at the side's then place the sole of your right foot on your left thigh slightly above the knee.

- Once you are balanced, bring your hands in front of you in the form of prayer position then raise them upwards.

- Hold the position for about 30 seconds then change the other leg.

## Benefits

- Improves balance of the body as well as strengthening the thighs, ankles, calves, legs and the spine.

## 8. Child Pose

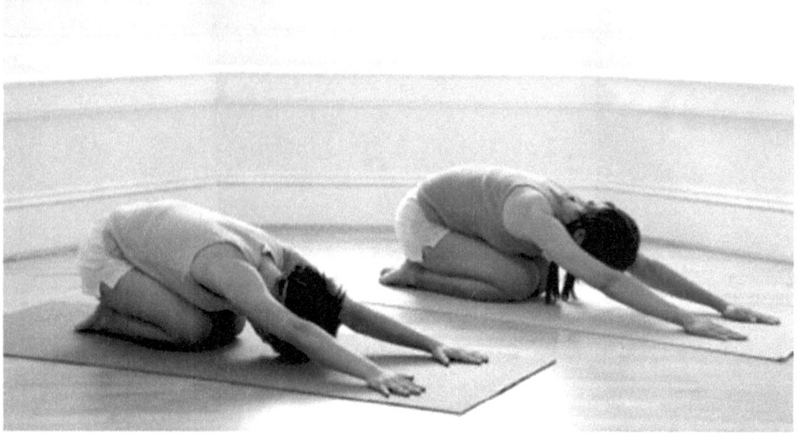

## Steps

- Place your palms down as you lean on your thighs as shown in the pose.

- Let your thighs stay as in the shown pose then exhale as you bring your chest closer to your knees and stretching your hands forward.

- Breathe gently as you hold on the posture for about 3 minutes

- Come back to the starting position then repeat the cycle 6 times or more.

## Benefits

- Cures back pains while also releasing tension, stress, and fatigue.

- Stretches the thighs, hips, and ankles while also relaxing front body muscles

## 9. Cobra pose

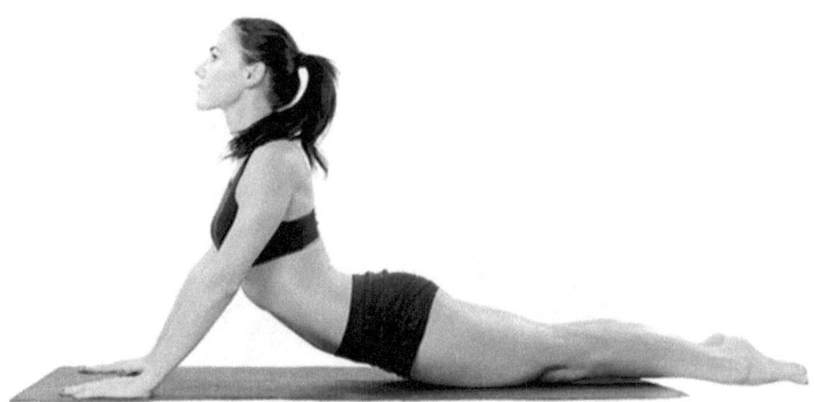

## Steps

- Lie down on your belly then take a deep breath as you raise your upper body and chest upwards as shown in the pose.

- Hold on the position for some time then exhale as you bring the upper part of your body to the ground.

- Repeat the cycle for about 5 times.

## Benefits

- Relieves conditions such as indigestion, constipation, and acidity.

- Reduces belly fat while also improving blood circulation

## 10. Butterfly pose

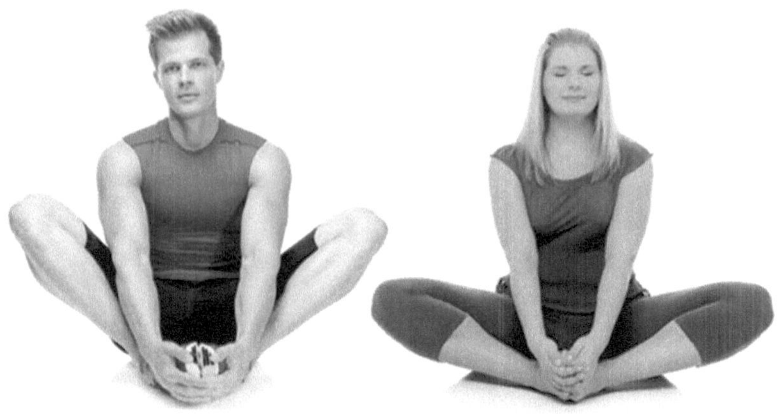

## Steps

- Sit on the floor straight with your spine erect then bend your knees and bring your feet as closer as you can.

- Try and ouch the soles of your feet as you hold with hands as shown in the pose.

- Flap like a butterfly by bringing your thighs up and down slowly for about 2 minutes

## Benefits

- Improves functioning of abdominal organs, the prostrate glands, kidneys and the bladder.

## 11. Quarter Dog

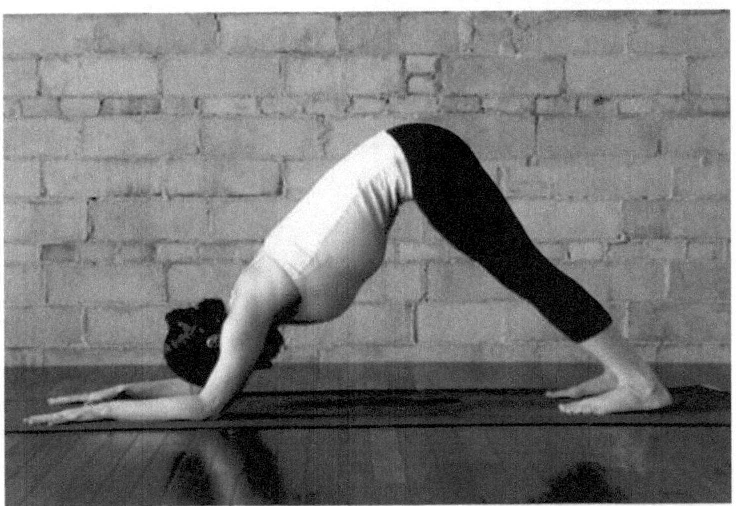

**Steps**

- Bend your hands and knees with your wrists underneath your shoulders and your knees beneath the hips.

- Inhale as you place your toes underneath your knees then exhale as you lift your hips as per the pose.

- Create a straight line between your elbows and the middle fingers.

- Straighten your fingers as you lower your arms and straighten your legs as you lower your heels towards the ground.

- Your heels should be wider than your toes. Relax your head between your arms as you direct your gaze towards your belly.

- Stay in the position as you hold your breath five times.

**Benefits**

- Stretches out the hamstrings, lower back, and calves.

- It also takes the weight off the hands and wrists.

## 12. Wheel Pose

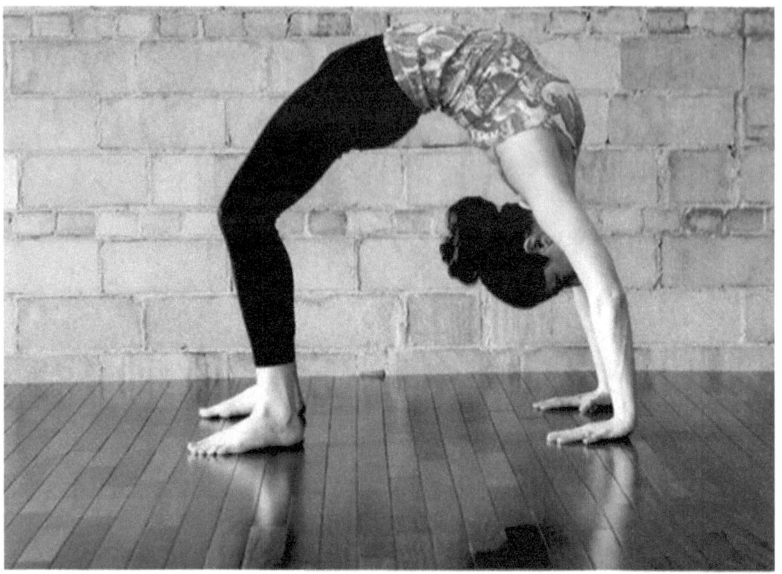

### Steps

- Lie on your back and you bend your knees with your feet placed on the ground. Bend your elbows then place the palms on the ground as shown in the pose above.

- Inhale and press your palms as you lift your head off the ground and exhale.

- Inhale deeply once in the pose as you try to walk with your hands and feet when closer together.

- Stay in the position as you take five deep breaths then slowly lower your body down. You can do the pose three times then relax.

### Benefits

- Increases flexibility and strengthens the spine and shoulders.

- Strengthens the upper body while also stretching the abs and quads making it ideal for runners.

## 13. Breathing Pose

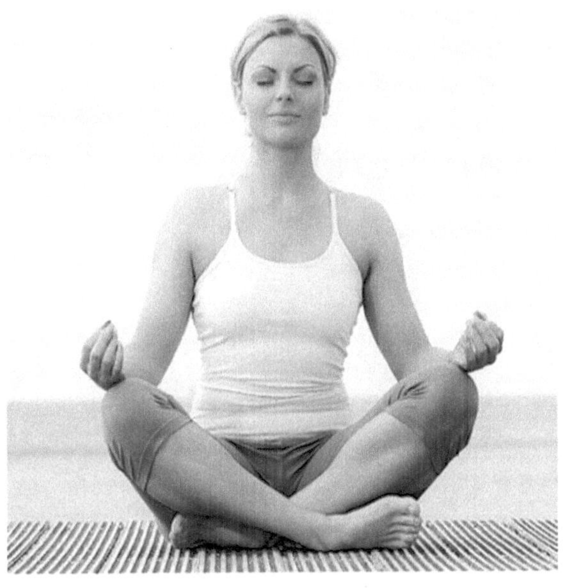

## Steps

- Sit on the mat with your back straight and head raised and focused

- Cross your legs as expressed in the pose as you rest your hands on your ankles.

- Stay in the position as you inhale and hold your breath to the count of seven then exhale.

- Exhale through your mouth while making a whoosh noise.

## Benefits

- Enhances the beauty and glow of the skin while enhancing the working of the lungs.

- Strengthens heart muscles and normalizes heart rate.

## 14. Headstand Pose

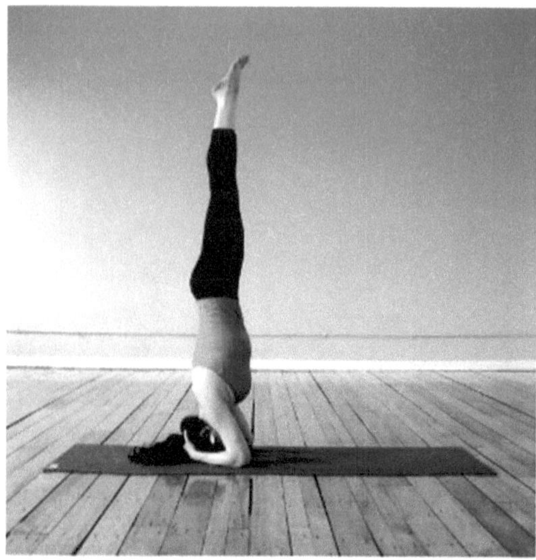

## Steps

- Place a mat on the ground then sit in a kneeling position.

- Bring your hands closer to your head with your elbows placed on the ground and your palms interlocked.

- Take deep breaths as you lift your body to a raised position as in the pose above.

- Begin by lifting one leg slowly up then follow up with another.

- It's advisable that you practice this pose with a professional help.

## Benefits

- Increases focus and relieve stress

- Improves blood flow to the eyes and the upper parts of the body

- Strengthens the shoulders and the arms

## 15. Corpse pose

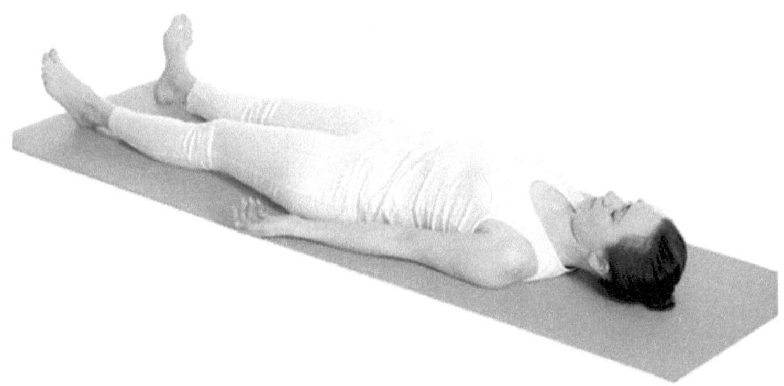

## Steps

- Lie down flat on the floor as you close your eyes

- Free your mind of all the negative thoughts as you relax completely

- Stand up straight with your leg apart then take quick breath with your face covered with the hands.

- Rub your facial skin, forehead and eyes then take ten deep breath.

- Repeat the process about 5 times.

## Benefits

- Relaxes the body and the mind and enables you to release the stress that you're carrying

- Enhances balance, flexibility, and strength of the body

- Peaceful association with death.

## 16. Shoulder stand pose

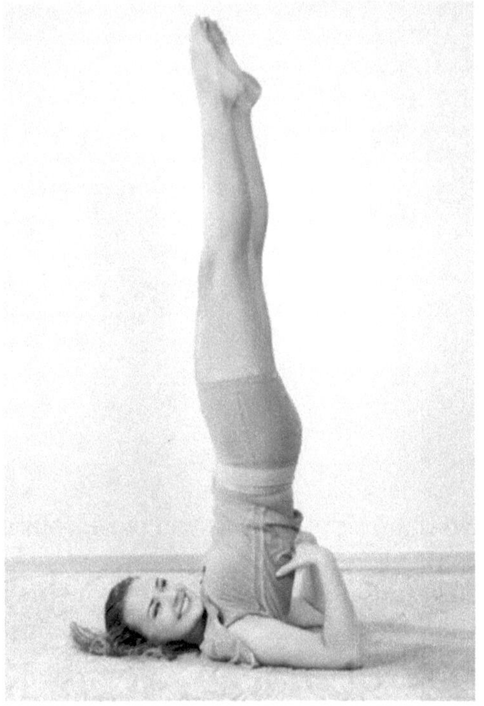

### Steps

- Keep your back straight as you raise your legs and your head to the opposite direction.

- You're likely to experience intense pressure on the shoulders.

- Use the palms to support your back and the lower body.

### Benefits

- Great exercise for a glowing face. It also relaxes the entire body and toughens the shoulders and upper parts of the body.

## 17. Twisted Seated Pose

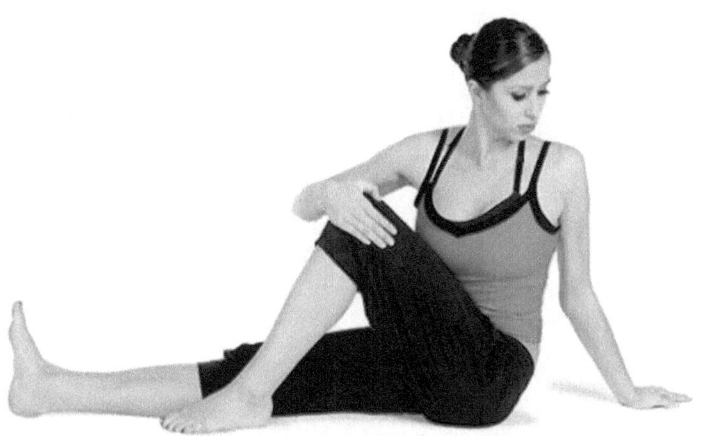

## Steps

- Sit on the floor cross-legged with your hands stretched to the sides.

- Breathe deeply as you shift your left hand to your right thigh then twist your torso.

- Exhale as you twist your body then hold on the position for about thirty seconds then repeat on the left side.

## Benefits

- Strengthens the spine while improving the overall well being

- Improves the digestive function

- Maintains the normal spinal rotation

- Relieves stress

## 18. Bow Pose

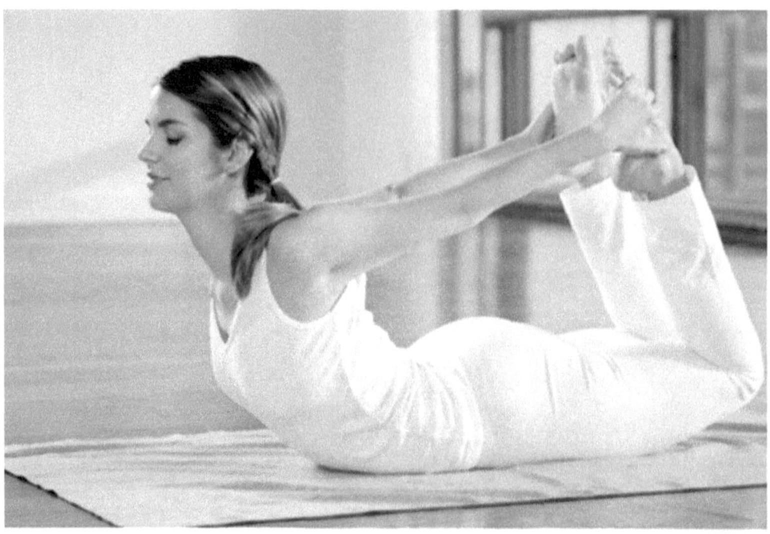

## Steps

- Lie on your stomach with your hands placed by your side. Your palms should face upwards.

- Bend your knees as you bring your heels closer to your buttocks.

- Stretch your hands as you hold your ankles then pull them together as your torso rises.

- Your body will then look like a bow. You should, however, breathe normally.

## Benefits

- Strengthens the back muscles, arms, legs, and abdomen.

- Tones the muscles and cultivates a supple and healthy spine.

- Improves the overall body posture.

## 19. Plough Pose

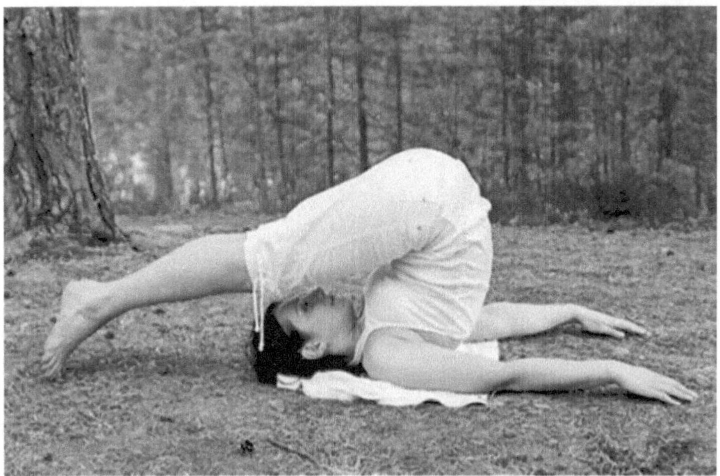

**Steps**

- Lie on the mat with your arms by your side then lift up your legs as a right angle gets formed between your upper and lower torso.

- Lift your hips slowly off the floor as you use your hands for balance.

- Lift your legs until they touch the flour beyond your head. It should look like the pose above; it should look more like an arch.

- Breathe normally then hold on the pose for about fifteen seconds then return to the normal position.

**Blessings**

- Calms the mind and stimulates the internal organs

- Activates the stretches, thyroid, the shoulders, and the hamstrings.

- Improves spines flexibility

## 20.   Sage Pose

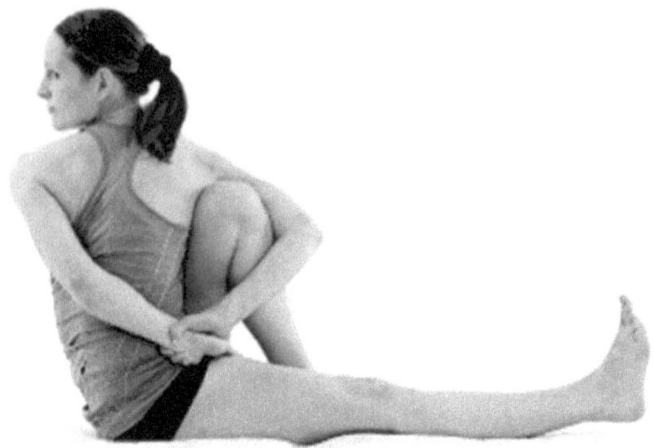

## Steps

- Sit on the flour then stretch your legs. Bend your right knee with your toes remaining flat on the ground and your feet closer to your pelvis.

- Bring the left knee closer to the chest and the toes should face upwards.

- Keep your spine straight as you stretch your arms on both sides.

- Take a deep breath as you twist your upper body from the waist towards the left slowly.

- Wrap the arms then slowly end your knees as you ensure they remain erect.

- Breathe normally during the process as your head and your shoulder face the opposite direction.

- Stay in the position for some time as you breathe normally then change to the other side.

## Benefits

- Enhances glowing of the skin while also stimulating the brain

- Stretches the shoulders and the spine

- Relieves backache and hip pain

## 21. Camel pose

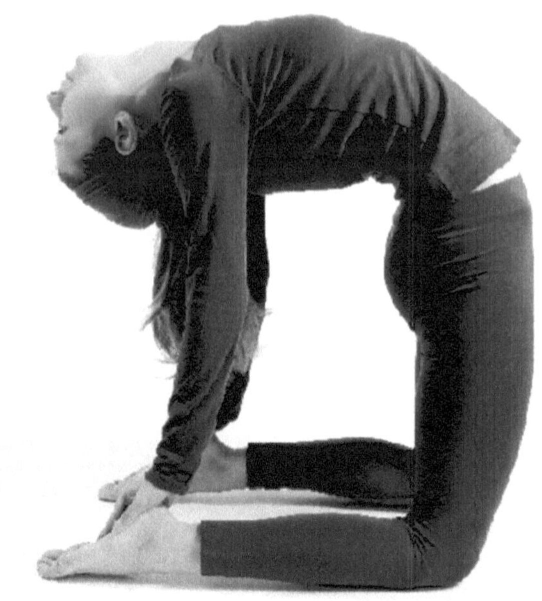

## Steps

- Kneel down then bend your back until your palms touch your feet.

- While in the pose, take deep breaths 7 times.

## Benefits

- Stretches the deep hip flexors and opens up the hips

- Stretches and strengthens the shoulder back

- Opens up the chest and improves respiration

- Relieves the lower back pain.

## 22. The wind Relieving Pose

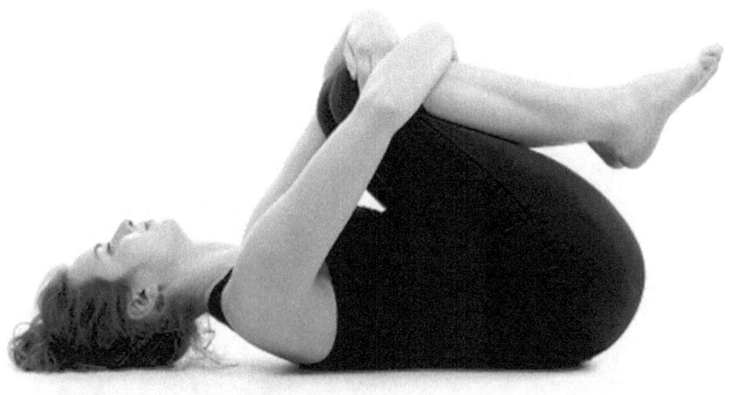

## Steps

- Lie on your back as you draw your knees closer to the chest

- Wrap your arms around your knees with your legs held closer together.

- Take deep breaths about 10 times while I the position.

## Benefits

- Stretches the muscles and speeds recovery from injury

- Releases tension on the lower back, thighs, and hips

- Relieves bloating, indigestion, acidity, and constipation

## 23. Warrior Lunge Twist

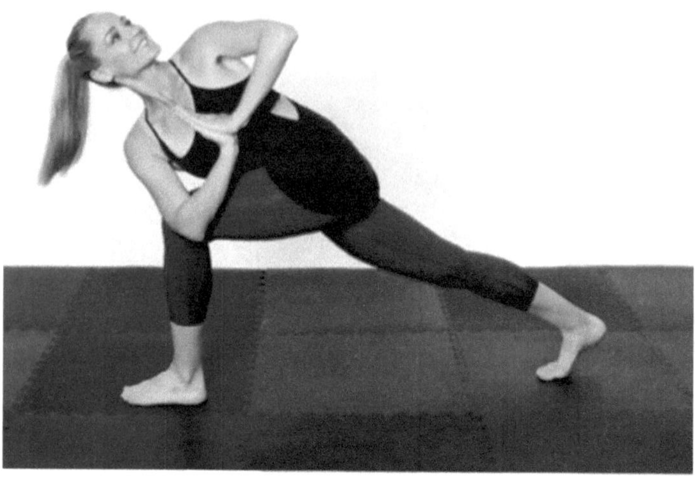

**Steps**

- Bring your hands into a prayer pose then stretch forward with your left leg as you bend your knee to about 90 degrees.

- Your back should be kept straight as you brace your abs tightly to your spine.

- Rotate the upper body to the left as you keep your spine straight and lean over on your left leg.

- Press the right elbow outside of your left leg then turn your head and look upwards over your left shoulder.

- Hold 10 deep breaths while in the position then repeat with the other side.

**Benefits**

- Stretches the hard to tone parts of the body.

- Enhances stability and flexibility of the body.

## 24. Warrior III

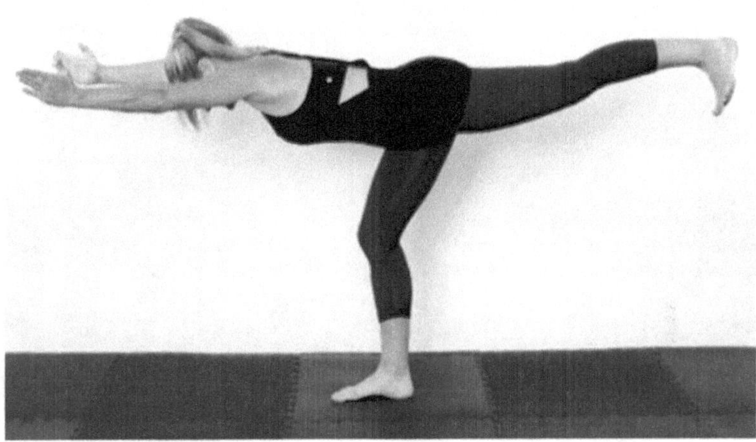

## Steps

- Shift your weight to the right foot then straighten your back to be parallel to the ground.

- Flex your left foot as you point your toes down.

- Stretch your arms in front of you so that your body is straight from your fingertips down to your back and heel.

- Stay in the position as you take 3 deep, long breaths then return slowly to standing as you repeat on the other side.

## Benefits

- Strengthens the legs while opening up the hips

- Improves circulation of blood and respiration while energizing the entire body

- Healing from injuries

## 25. Extended Boat Pose

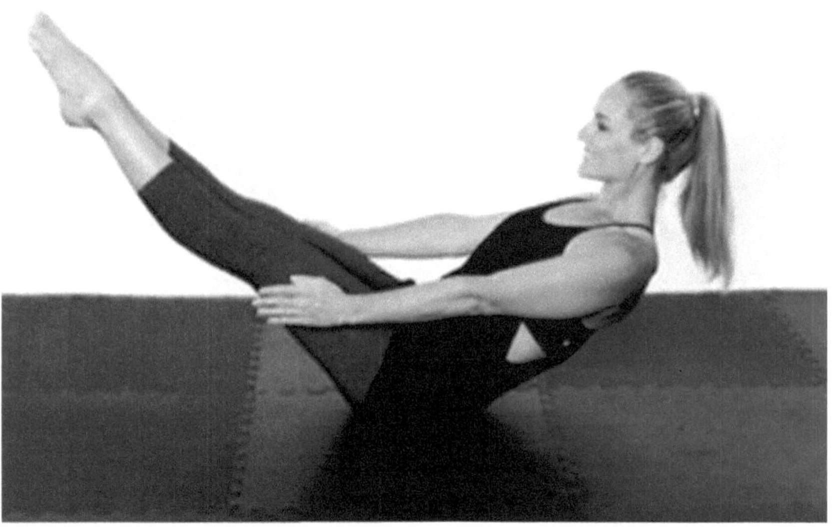

### Steps

- Sit on your hips as you stretch your legs in front of you. Place your hands behind the hips then lean your back slightly as you raise your legs above the floor while holding your stomach in.

- Stretch both the arms to the sides of your thigh then lower your legs to about 45 degrees or until the body are in V shape.

- Take 10 deep and long breaths while in the position.

### Benefits

- Builds your core strength and enhances endurance.

- Relieves gas and bloating

- Strengthens the back and the abdomen

## 26.Sliding Table

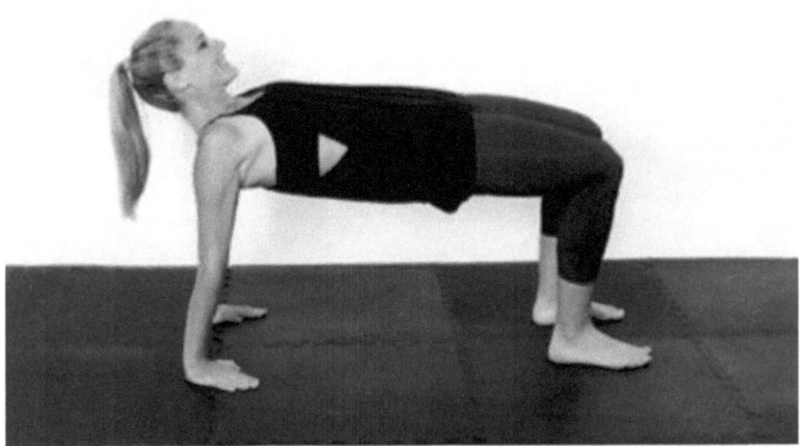

## Steps

- Sit on the flour with your knees bent and your feet flat on the flour and hip wide.

- Place your hands behind the hips with your fingertips facing your body slightly.

- Lift your hips to appear in a table top position as in the pose.

- Extend your legs then push the hips back until your pelvis is behind the hips.

- Hold on the position for some time then you can repeat up to 10 times.

## Benefits

- Stretches the back and the upper body, chest, and spine

- Strengthens the muscles around the spine

### 27. Stacked side Plank

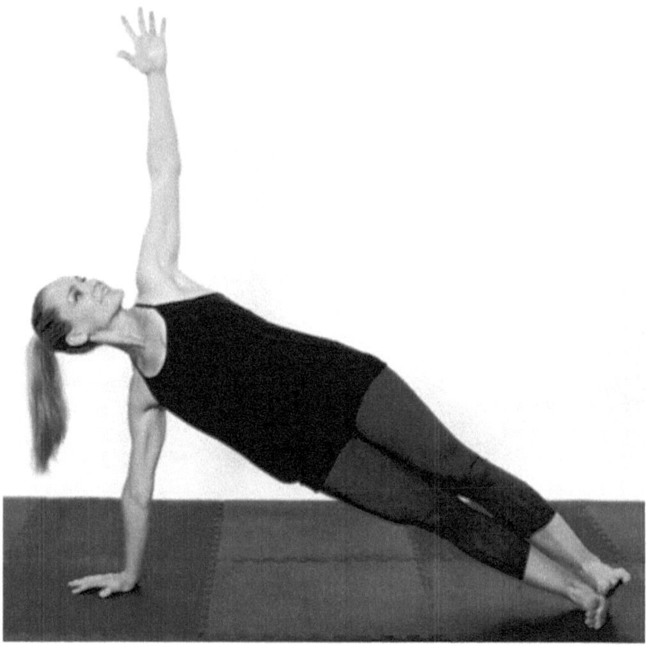

### Steps

- Lie on your right side as you straighten your knees.

- Place your right hand on the shoulder as you raise your hips off the floor as your body forms into a straight line right from your ankles to the shoulders.

- Stretch your arms towards the ceiling as you breathe deeply for the time of the exercise.

- Stay in the position for about 60 seconds then lower and repeat with the other side.

### Benefits

- Strengthens the entire body and the abdominal area.

## 28.Lotus Hip Lift

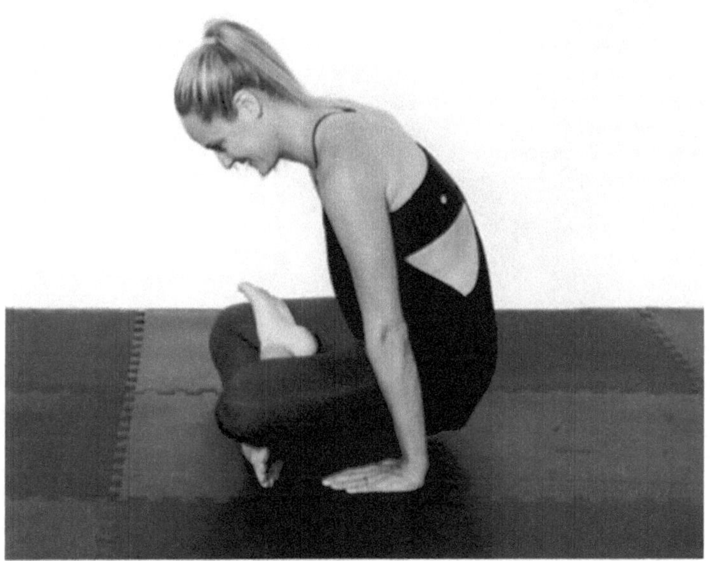

## Steps

- Sit on the floor with crossed legs and pressed palms outside the hips.

- The fingertips should face forward as you brace your abs and press your arms down.

- Lift your hips off the flour then hold in the position for about 3 counts.

- Lower then repeat a few times.

## Benefits

- Straightens the spine while enhancing awareness and attentiveness

- Calms the brain and relieves stress

## 29.Side Fierce

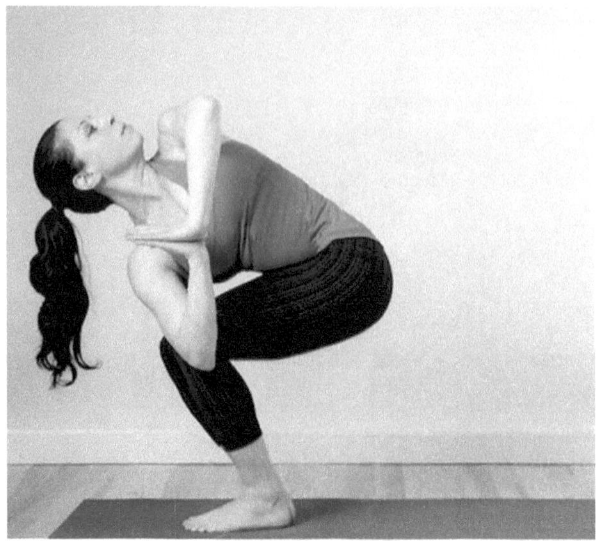

## Steps

- Stand on the floor with both feet close together

- Bend your knees as you squat into fierce pose then rotate your torso and cross the right elbow over to the outside of the right thigh.

- Press closer to your arm as if to lift the torso then pull the right hip back for your knees to line and keep the weight back to your heels.

- Hold onto the position as you take five deep breaths while gazing over your left shoulder.

## Benefits

- Strengthens the shoulders, arms, and wrists

- Strengthens the legs and improves balance

- Improves concentration and focus

## 30.     Arching three legged dog

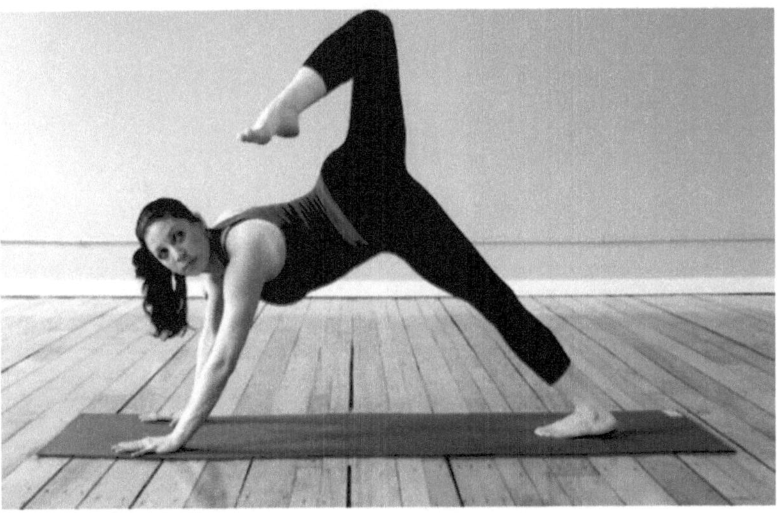

## Steps

- From the side, fierce arise into the fierce pose then take the pose of a downward facing dog.

- Place both feet together as you leave the left heel on the mat and raise the right leg upwards then bend the knee.

- Squeeze the right heel towards your hip as you lift your knee high.

- Lift our head up then turn and look over the left shoulder and the arching spine.

- Hold onto the position as you take a few breaths while keeping your belly still as you breathe through the chest.

## Benefits

- Stretches and strengthens the entire body

- Rejuvenates the brain

### 31. Wide legged Forward Bend

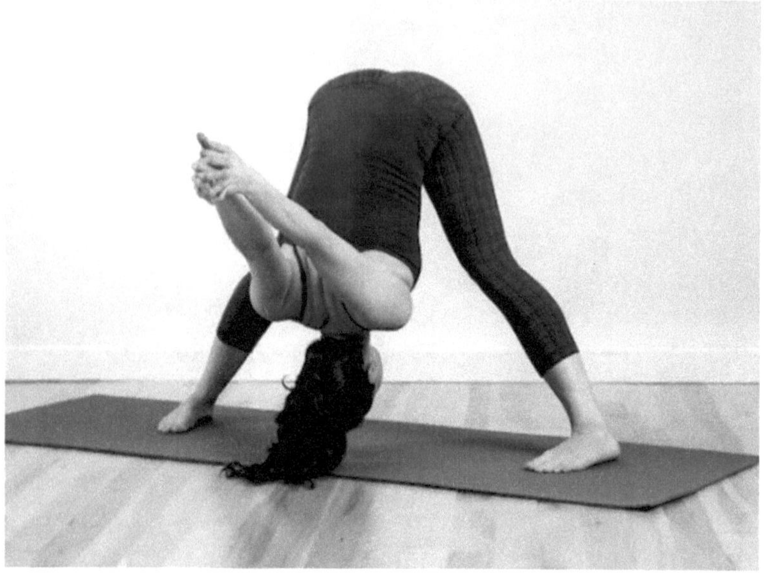

## Steps

- Stand on your feet at 5 ft apart with the heels facing outwards.

- Stand tall as you interlace your hands behind you and pressing your palms together.

- Inhale deeply as you fold at your waist while lowering and stretching your hand.

- Stretch your back straight as you take 5 deep breaths.

- Engage the legs as you slowly rise up.

## Benefits

- Opening of tight hamstrings

- Enhances blood circulation all through the body.

- Enhances digestion

## 32. Open side fierce

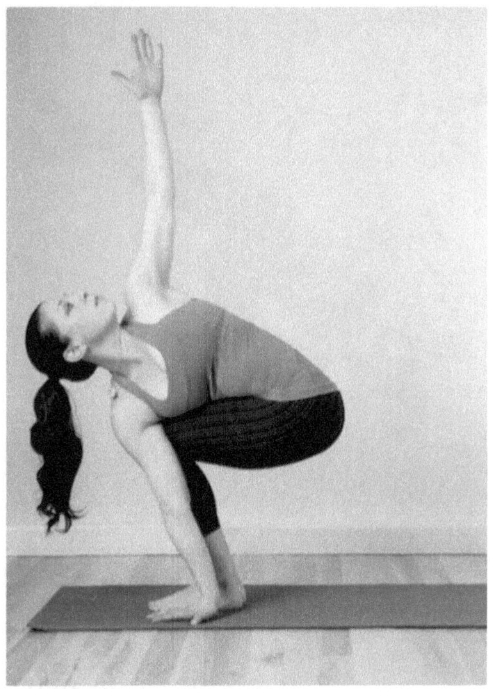

**Steps**

- Stand with both your feet together then bend your knees and squat as you come to a fierce pose.

- Cross your right elbow over to your left thigh as you place your right palm on the floor next to your foot.

- Stretch your left arm towards the ceiling straight as you shift your shoulder and gaze at the lifted palm.

- Ensure that the knees are parallel as you hold in the position for five deep breaths then change to the right side.

**Benefits**

- Strengthens lower legs and aids digestion

- Stimulates removal of waste from the body.

## 33. Half Moon

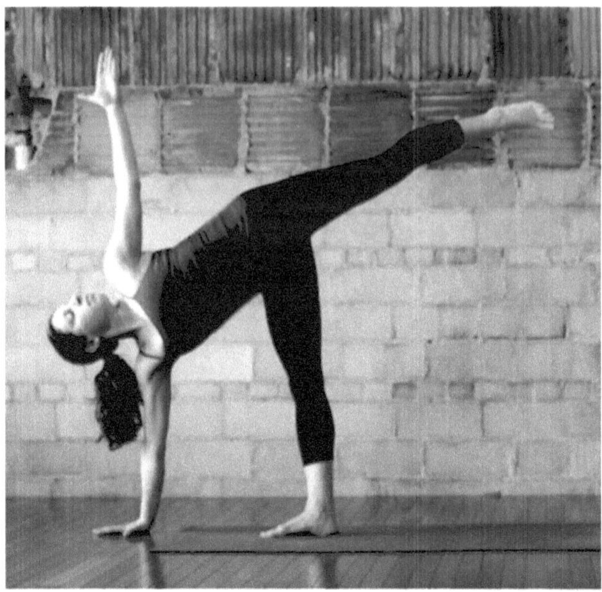

## Steps

- Start with downward facing dog position then step forward with your right foot and rise into warrior 1 position.

- Open your chest, arms and hips then place your hand on the left hip as you stretch your arm straight out.

- Shift weight on the right foot as you lift your left foot

- Place your right palm on the ground flat under your shoulder then bend the right knee.

- Raise your left arm up straight then look towards the raised arm.

- Hold the position for five breaths then try the half moon pose on the left side.

## Benefits

- Strengthens the body while reducing the back fat

- Strengthens the groins, hamstrings and the calves.

## 34. Extended table top

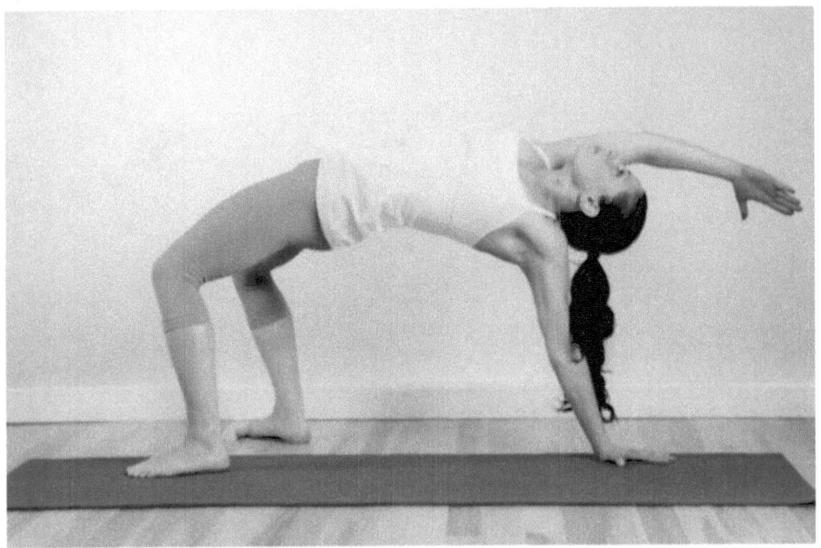

## Steps

- Place your feet on the floor as you also lower your left hand on the floor.

- Raise your right arm in the air. It should be like rotating your body to 180 degrees as your belly faces upwards.

- Your feet should be wide apart and parallel to each other.

- Hold on the position for five deep breaths as you gaze at the extended hands or towards the ceiling.

## Benefits

- Increases flexibility by opening the front of your body.

- It also tones your body

## 35. Extended wide squat

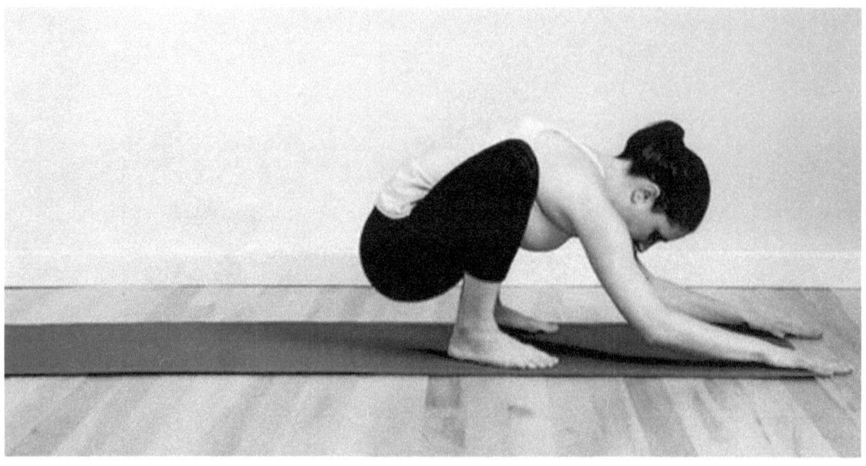

## Steps

- Squat with your legs slightly apart. Place your hands on the floor then lean as if pressing your belly towards the floor.

- Relax your head as you lower it towards the floor.

## Benefits

- Stretches and relaxes the hips and the spine.

- Calms the head and the arms.

- Strengthens the abdominal areas.

## 36. Happy Baby Pose

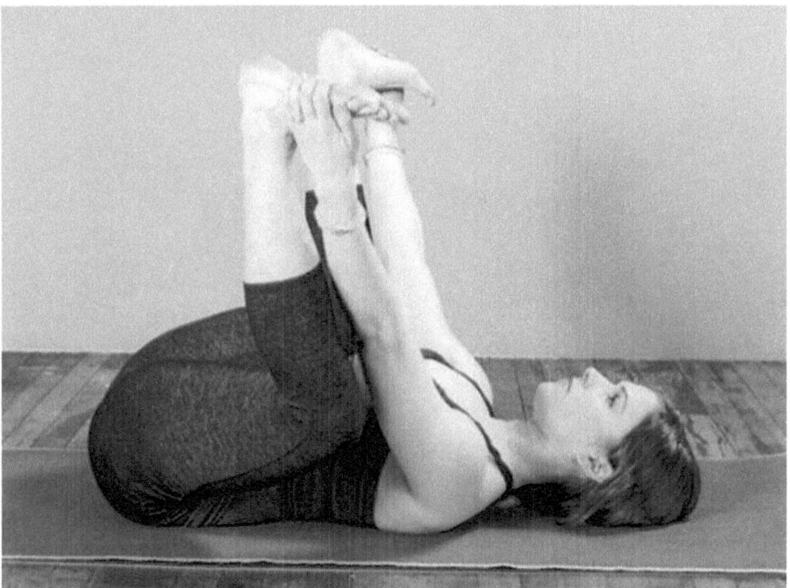

## Steps

- Lie on a mat and pull your knees closer to the chest.

- Place your hands on your feet as you open your knees to be wider than your torso.

- Press your feet into the hands as you pull down your feet so as to create resistance.

- Breathe deeply as you hold the breath for about 30 seconds.

## Benefits

- Opens up the hips, the inner thighs, and the groin

- Stretches the hamstrings and relieves the lower back pain

- Soothes and stretches the spine

- Relieves fatigue and stress

## 37. Reclining Hero Pose

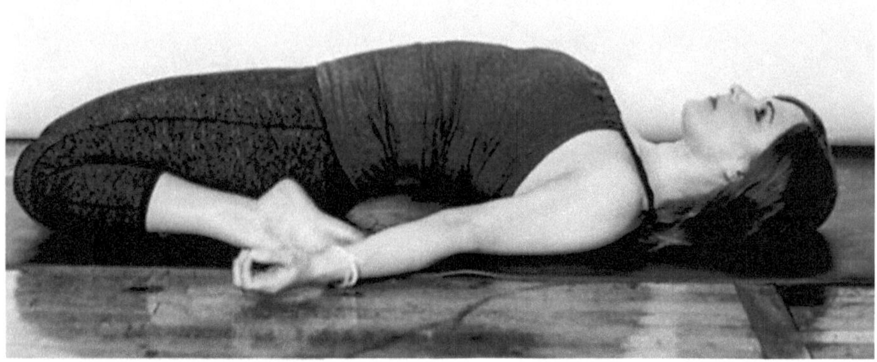

## Steps

- Kneel on the mat with your thighs in a perpendicular to the floor and the top of the feet facing down.

- Slide your feet apart to be wider than the hips then press your feet on the mat.

- Sit down slowly at your feet then use your hands t turn the top of your thighs inwards.

- Lean back to your arms as you lower your torso to the floor.

- Hold onto the position for about 30 seconds.

## Benefits

- Helps and relieves the tired legs

- Improves digestion and the mental discomfort

- Strengthens the arches of the feet

## 38. Half Pigeon

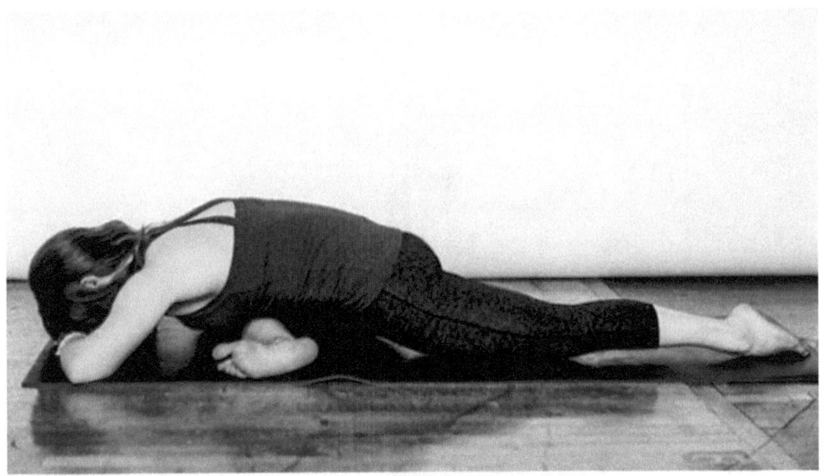

## Steps

- Start with your right leg forward and the right knee over the right ankle with the back of the leg straight.

- Stretch the right foot towards the left hand then drop your right shin and your thigh on the floor as you keep the right knee with the right hip.

- Let your left leg rest on the floor with the top of your foot facing down.

- Hold on the position as you breathe normally for about 30 seconds then alternate to the opposite side.

## Benefits

- Stimulates the internal organs while also stretching deep glutes

- Stretches the groins and the abdominal muscles

## 39. Crescent Lunge

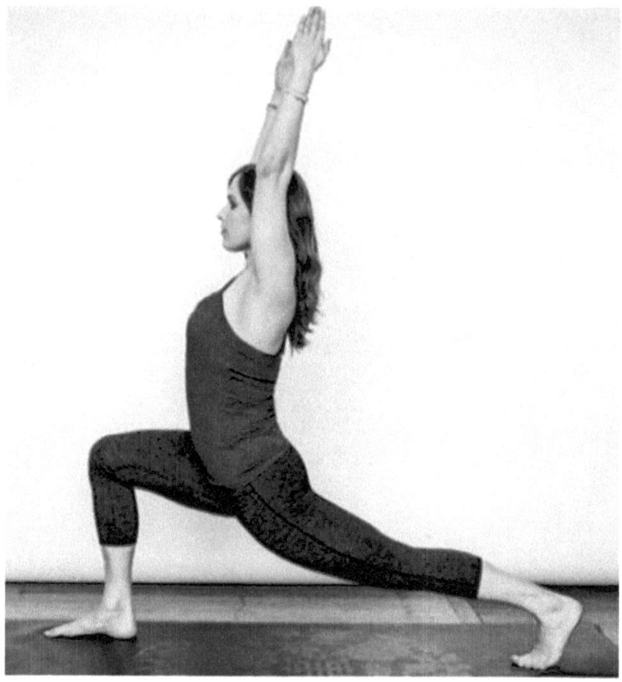

## Steps

- Begin in a low lunge as you straighten your back leg with your heels raised.

- Hold onto the position for about 30 seconds then repeat with the opposite side.

## Benefits

- Stretches the groins, legs and the hip flexors

- Strengthens and tones the thighs, hips and the butt.

- Enhances flexibility and stability

## 40.    Killer Praying Mantis

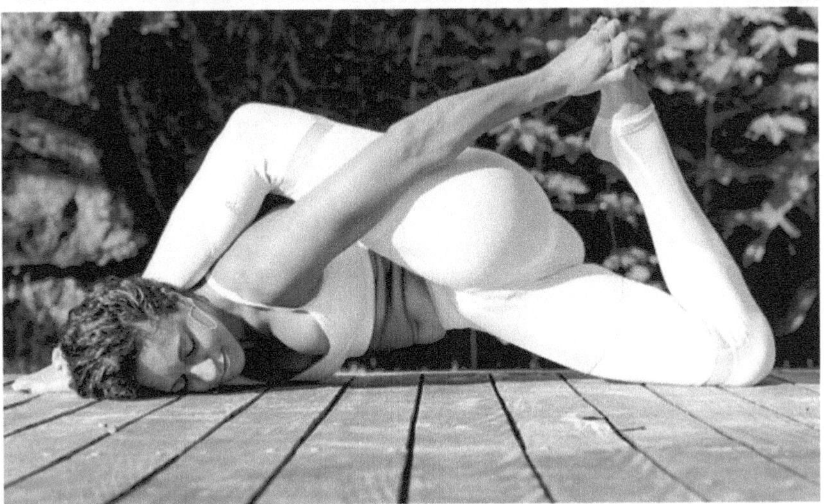

## Steps

- Lie on the floor then raise your left leg above your head as in the pose.

- Fold your right thighs then raise your legs straight as you stretch your left hand to hold your right feet.

- Bring your left leg closer to your neck with your right hands holding on the right leg

- Take deep breaths six times while in the position then relax and change to the other side.

## Benefits

- Strengthens muscles in the entire body while opening up the hips.

- Enhances the functioning of the inner organs and blood circulation

## 41. Headstand with lotus legs

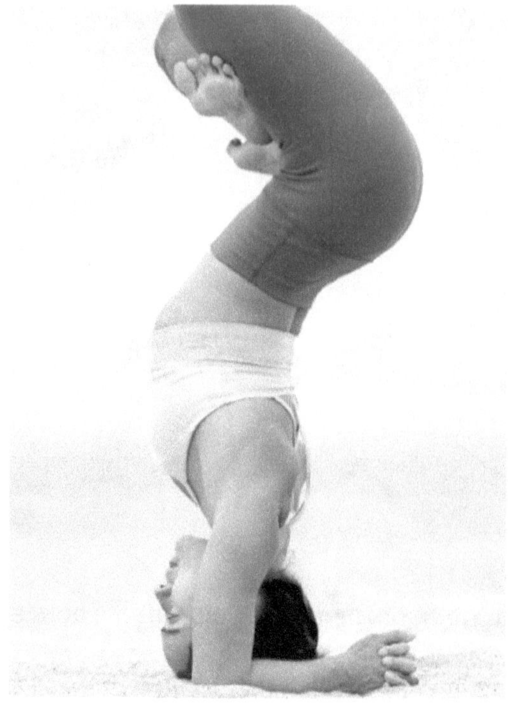

## Steps

- Place your head on the floor then raise your legs towards the ceiling.

- Let your arms rest outside your head and your hands held together behind your head.

- Bend your thighs and your legs folded and drawn closer to the hips as in the pose above.

- Take five deep long breaths while in the position.

## Benefits

- Increased blood flows to the brain while addressing nervous related issues.

- Improves memory and relieves stress

## 42.One Arm Compass

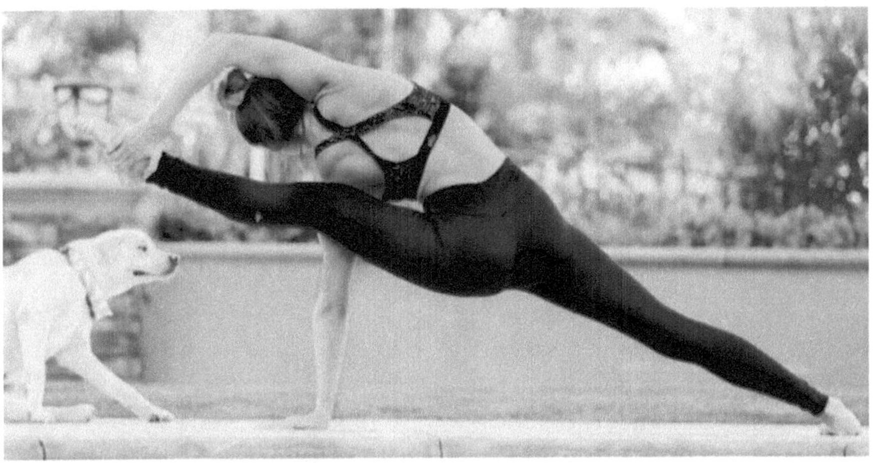

## Steps

- Begin by placing standing on the floor with your feet five feet wide and both your hands pressing on the ground.

- Lift your left leg off the ground as you transfer the body weight to your left hand and right leg.

- Stretch your right hand up above your head then grab your left leg as shown in the pose

- Stay in the position as you take 10 deep breaths

## Benefits

- Enhances strength, balance, and flexibility of the entire body.

- Strengthens the spine, hamstring and improved blood circulation

## 43. Bound side crow

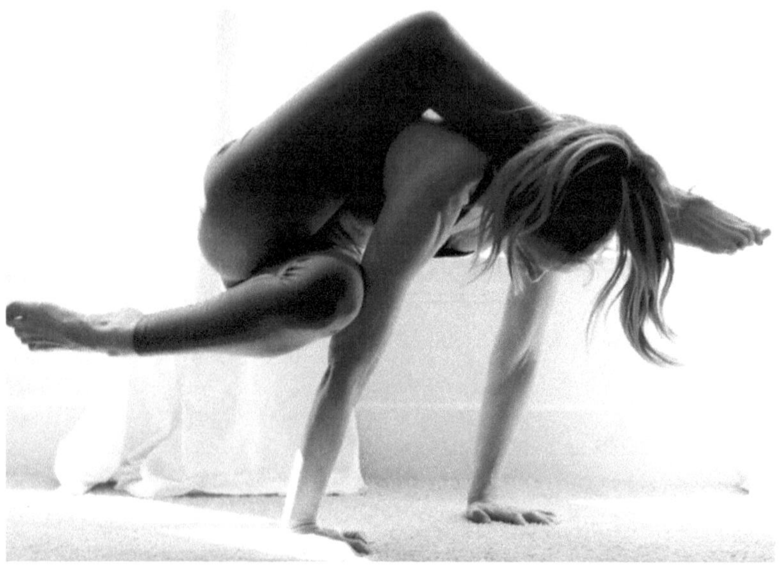

## Steps

- Bend your knees to half squat with your thighs parallel to the floor. Take the left elbow outside the thigh as you twist your torso to the right

- Place your right leg above your neck as you bend your left leg with your thighs leaning on your right arm

- Take a deep breath while in the position then relax and change to the other side.

## Benefits

- Strengthens the wrists and arms

- Tones the spine and the belly

- Improves balance of the body

## 44. Arms and a twist

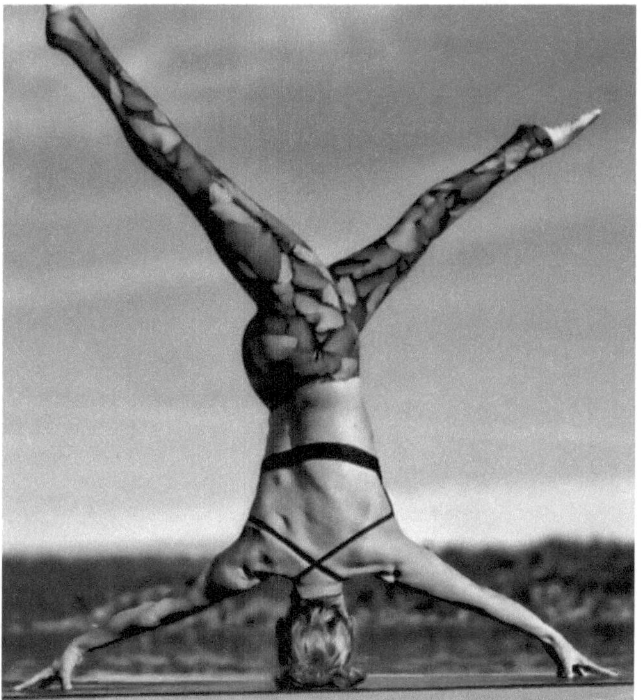

## Steps

- Place your head on the floor with hands wide apart and pressed on the ground.

- Stretch your legs towards the ceiling then twist your legs as shown in the pose above.

- Stay I the position as you take deep long breaths about five times

## Benefits

- Improves blood flow to the brain while strengthening the upper body muscles.

- Enhances stability and balance of the body.

## 45. Mermaid in Low Lunge

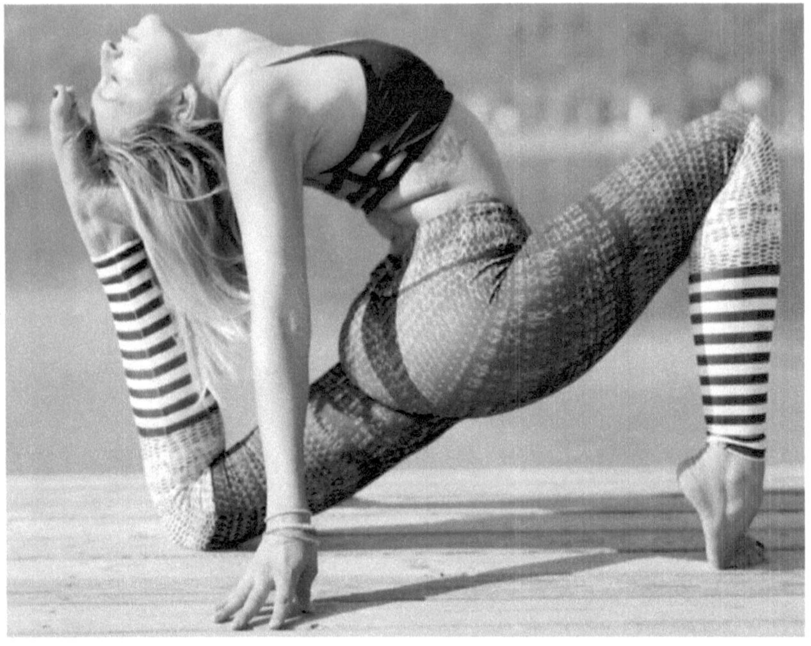

**Steps**

- Take the downward facing dog position as you inhale and lift your right leg and step it between your hands. The right ankle should be placed directly under the knee.

- Lower your back as you raise your left knee and your head resting on your leg as shown n the pose.

- Lengthen your torso upright as you relax the shoulders. Hold several breaths while in the position then change to the left side.

**Benefits**

- Cultivates strength and fluidity. Increases strength, stability, and flexibility.

- Ideal for people who sit a lot.

## 46.Eagle Pose

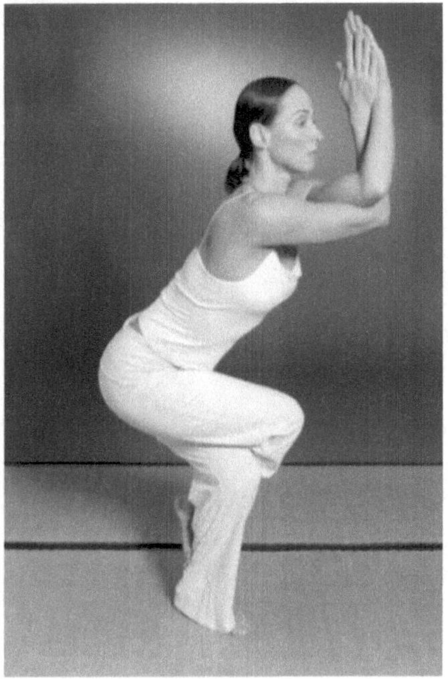

## Steps

- Begin by standing in mountain pose with your arms at the sides then bend the knees

- Stretch your arms in front of the body as you also bend your elbows and raise your forearms to be perpendicular to the floor

- Cross your thighs with your right leg foot placed behind the left one.

- Raise your head and gaze straight as you take several deep breaths then change to the other side.

## Benefits

- Strengthens the arms, knees, legs and the joints.

- Helps in creating space between the shoulder blades.

## 47. Cat Pose

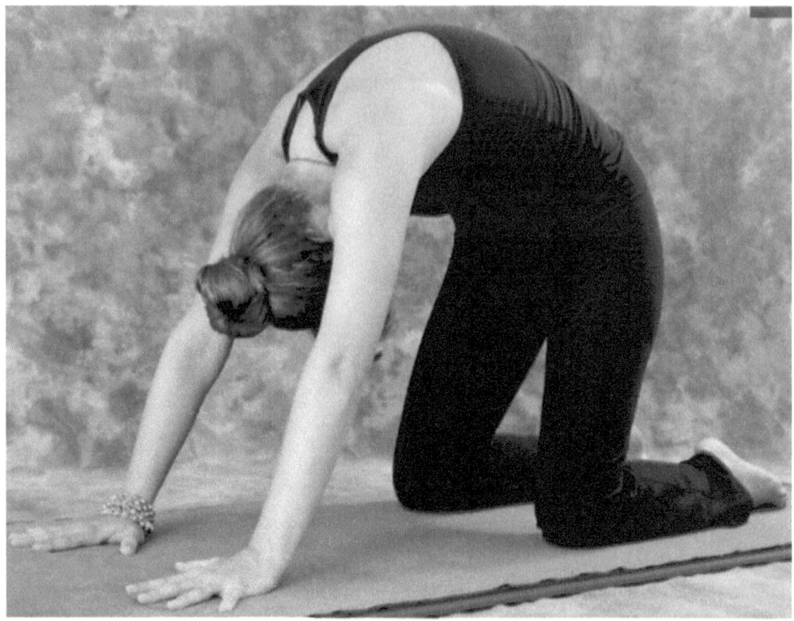

## Steps

- Breathe in as you bend forward from the hips then place your palms on the floor and your fingers with hands apart.

- Bring your forward close to the knees as you keep the knees straight.

- Stay in the position as you take deep breaths ten times.

## Benefits

- Improves body posture and balance

- Stretches and strengthens the spine and the neck.

- Stretches the hips, the back, and the abdomen while increasing coordination.

- Massages and stimulates belly organs.

## 48.  Warrior 11

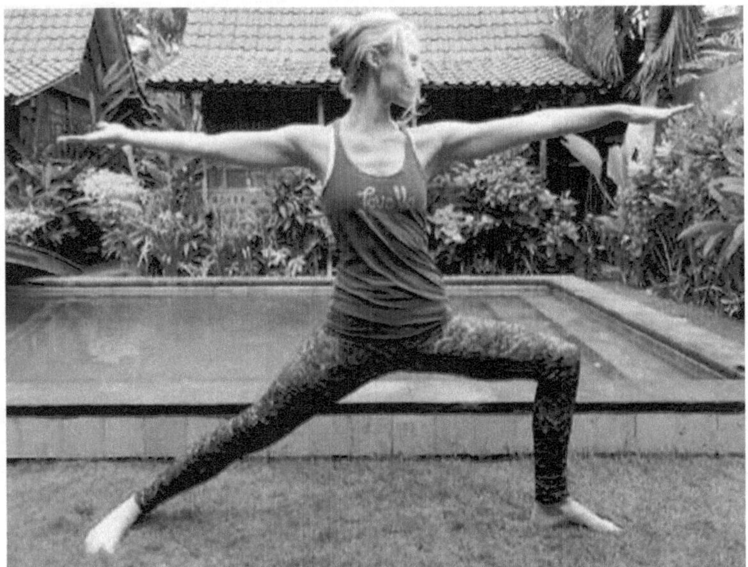

## Steps

- Stand straight with the legs apart then inhale as you raise your and stretch both your hands

- Stretch your legs then bend your right knee as you keep your arms and shoulders straight.

- Inhale as you twist to the front then exhale as you twist to the right side.

- Repeat it several times.

## Benefits

- Strengthens the legs and opens the hips and the chest

- Enhances level of concentration, balance, and stability

- Improves blood circulation and energizes the entire body

## 49.Reversed Child's pose

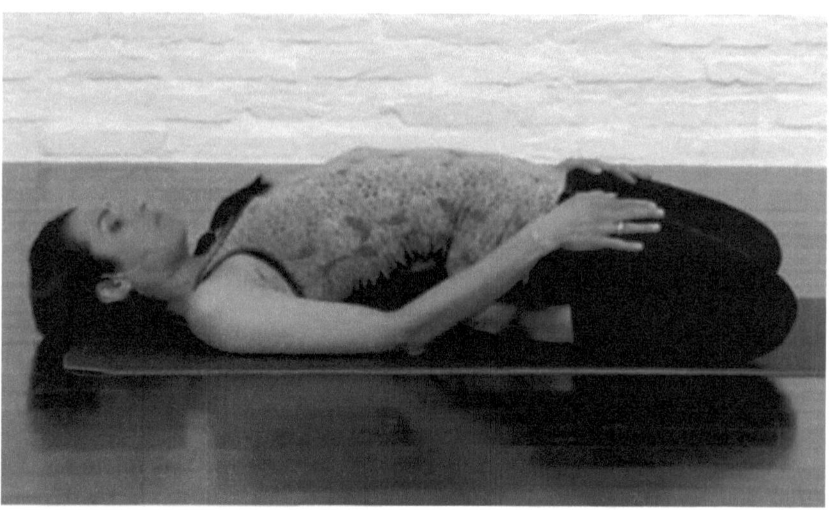

## Steps

- Begin by lying on the floor then bending your knees below your hips as in the pose above.

- Your hips should rest on your legs as you place your arms on the thighs

- Raise your torso as your head and shoulders rest on the floor.

- Take several deep breaths as you stay in the position.

## Benefits

- Speeds up digestion while also strengthening the thigh muscles and the calves

## 50. Thread the Needle

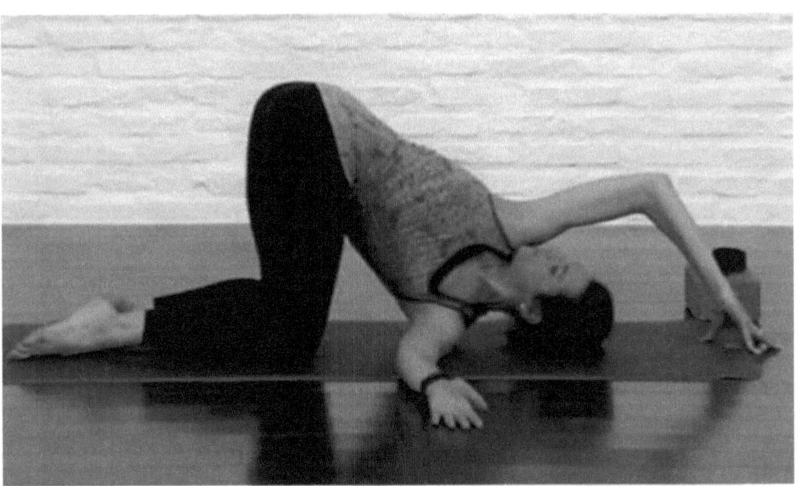

## Steps

- Kneel on the floor as you twist your torso with your head on the floor.

- Let your left hand rest freely on the floor as you transfer pressure to your left hand with your fingers pressing the floor.

- Take deep breaths as you stay in the position for some time.

## Benefits

- Strengthens the upper body and the neck muscles.

- Enhances stability and strength

## 51. Handstand Scorpion

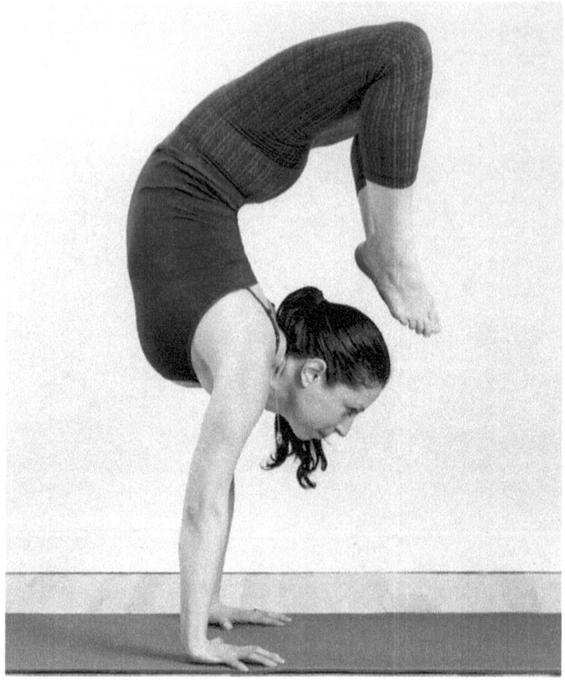

### Steps

- Start with a downward dog pose then raise your legs up and stretch your hips apart.

- Stretch your legs as you also raise your head with both your palms on the floor firmly

- Take deep breaths while I the position with your head raised and eyes fixed on the floor

### Benefits

- Stretches the chest, neck, abs, and spine.

- Strengthens the arms the back and the shoulders

- Stimulates the abdominal organs and the lungs.

- Increases fertility and stimulates the reproductive organs.

## 52. King Pigeon Pose

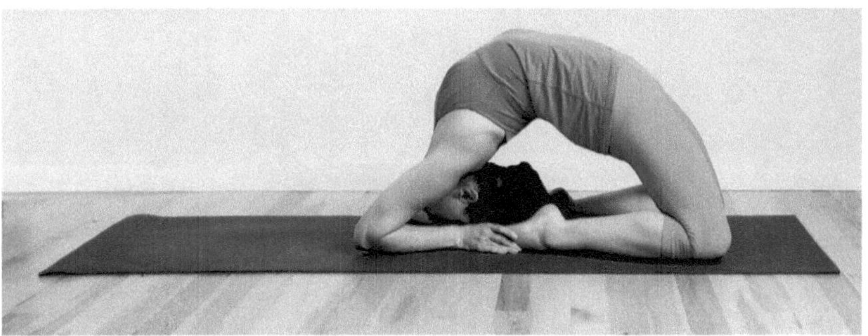

## Steps

- Start with your legs on the floor beneath your hips and your hips raised

- Bend your torso until your face faces the floor as in the pose with your hands next to your head.

- Take several deep breaths while in the position

## Benefits

- Stretches the groins, abdomen, the thighs and the rest of the body

## 53. Half Lotus Crow

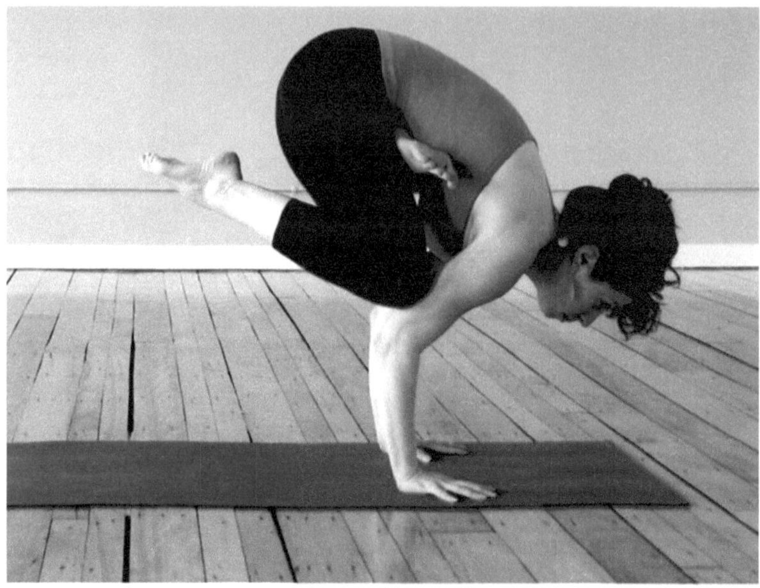

## Steps

- Begin with the half lotus spinal twist then release your hands and bring the torso closer to the center.

- Place your palms in front of you as your feet are kept in half lotus

- Place your knees as high onto your triceps as you can

- Spread the weight to your hands as you lift the right foot off the floor.

- Hold the body in the position for five breaths.

## Benefits

- Strengthens the back while also stretching the ankles, knees, thighs and the hips

- Reduces stress, increases stability and strengthens the spine.

## 54. Iron Cross Headstand

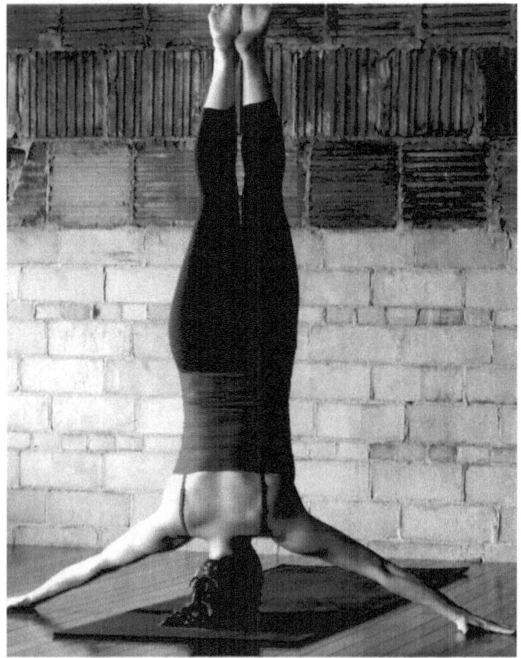

## Steps

- Start with a head stand position then stretch your hands with both your palms placed on the floor.

- Bend your legs for body stability then stretch your legs straight towards the ceiling

- Move your arms so that your head stays in the middle

- Hold onto the position as you take five deep breaths.

## Benefits

- Enhances blood circulation to the brain and upper parts of the body.

- Strengthens the upper body muscles and enhances balance and stability.

## 55. Scorpion with broken tail

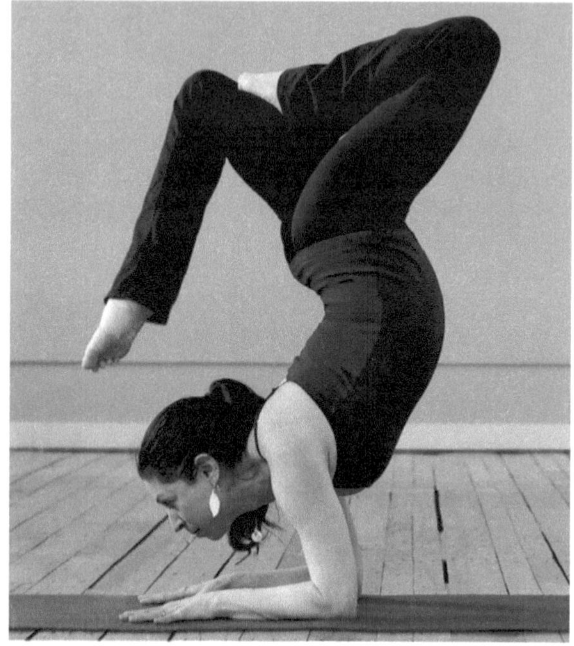

**Steps**

- Start off in quarter dog position with elbows on the ground

- Lift the right leg up as you keep the left foot on the ground.

- Kick the right leg over the head and follow with your left leg.

- Bend your right knee as you bring the foot towards the head

- Bend the left knee as you place the feet on the right knee.

- Hold on to the position as you take five deep breaths.

**Benefits**

- Enhances blood circulation n the body

- Strengthens the arms and the shoulders.

- Relaxes and balances the body

## 56. Chakra bond pose

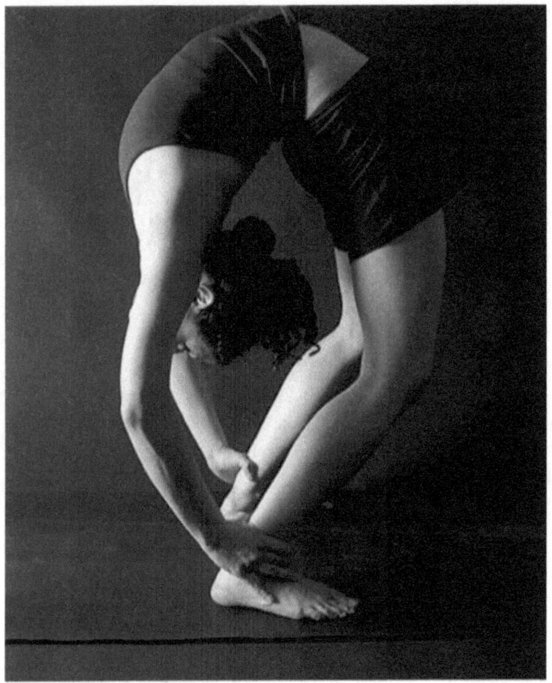

## Steps

- Begin in a standing position with your legs apart then bend backward until your hands touch both your heels.

- Bend your knees slightly as you bring your head right below your hips and between your legs as shown in the pose. Your hands and the feet should be in a parallel position.

- Hold onto the position as you take breath several times.

## Benefits

- Alleviates stress and revitalizes the body

- Enhances stability and strengthens the spine

## 57. Big toe bow

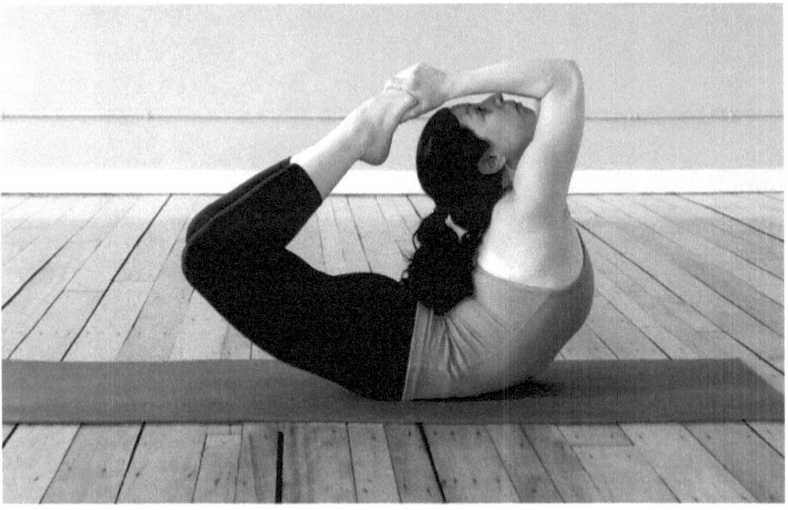

## Steps

- Lie flat on your belly as you press it on the floor then bend your knees and stretch your hands to grab both your feet.

- Get a firm hold of feet then try to pull it as high as possible as you shift your weight forward with your head raised.

- Hold onto the position as you take five deep breaths.

- You can repeat again or relax in a child's pose.

## Benefits

- Increases flexibility in the back and the spine

- Stretches the shoulders, the chest and improves digestion.

## 58.Sleeping yogi

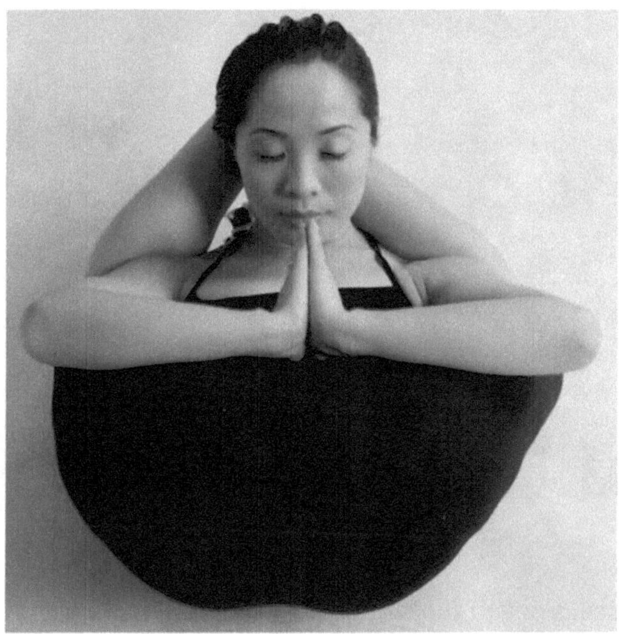

## Steps

- Begin with ling flat on the back as you bend both of the knees and hold onto edges of your feet with your hands

- Keep the arms outside the legs as you use the upper part of the body strength to press both your knees under the armpits.

- Avoid tensing your shoulders and the chest

- Stay in the position as you take five deep breaths.

## Benefits

- Stretches the lower back and the hamstrings.

- Enhances flexibility of the hips and the back.

- Increases sexual vitality.

## 59. Humming Bird

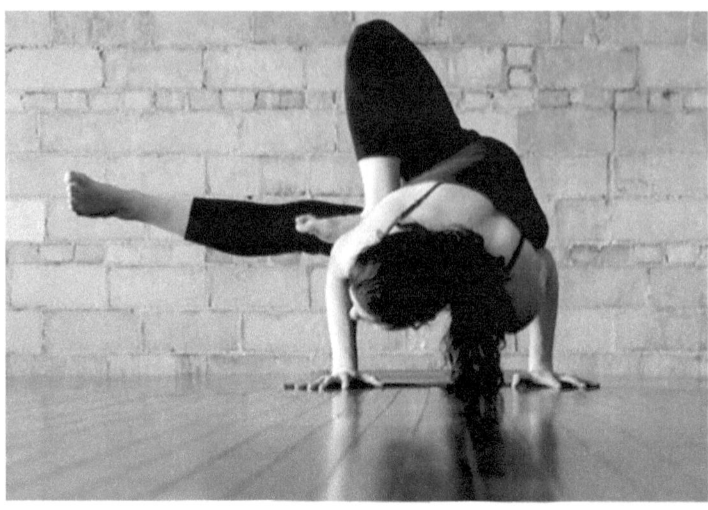

## Steps

- Begin in a mountain pose as you shift the weight to the left leg and cross the right leg above your knee. Your shin should be parallel to the floor

- Bend the left knee to 90 degrees angle as you twist your upper body to the right.

- Place the arch of the right foot closer to the right armpit then get the foot high for greater stability.

- Let your palms stay on the floor as your weight is transferred to the arms then extend the left leg.

- Hold onto the position for 10 breaths before placing your feet on the floor.

- Repeat with the other side.

## Benefits

- Strengthens the abdominal muscles, the spine, shoulders, and the arms.

- Relieves tension in the back while relaxing the entire body.

## 60.    Peacock Variation

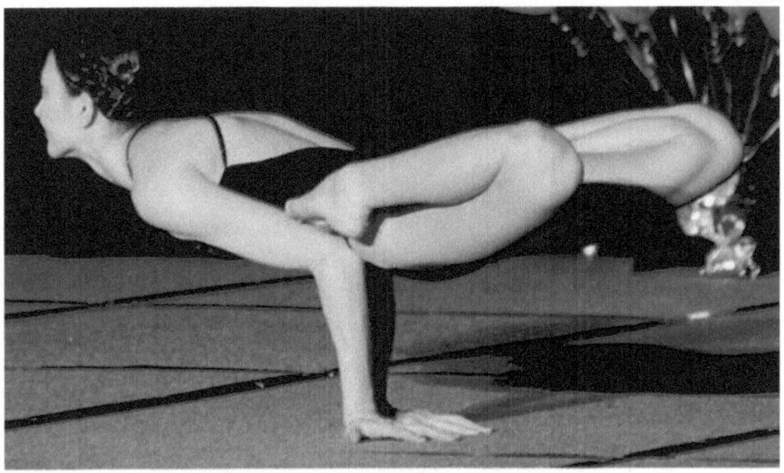

## Steps

- Begin in a kneeling position then place the palms on the floor with your fingers facing the direction of the knees.

- Transfer the weight of the body to your hands as you bend your feet with your legs resting on your hips.

- Raise your head and focus straight.

- Hold onto the position as you take between 5 – 10 breaths.

## Benefits

- Strengthens the heart muscles, the back, hips, hamstrings, and other body parts.

- Increases body coordination and balance

- Increases focus and concentration.

## 61. Firefly B

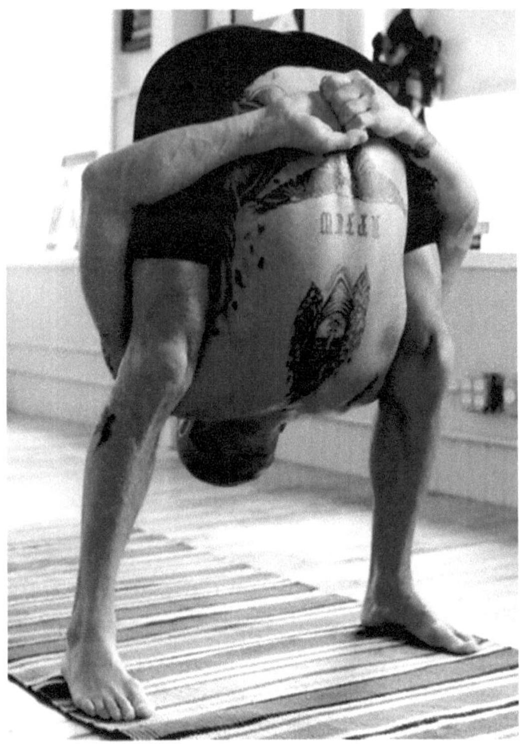

## Steps

- Stand in a mountain position then bend until your entire back is between your legs and your head below your hips.

- Stretch up your hands around your thighs then hold the hands together behind your back.

- Hold onto the position as you take between 5 – 10 breaths.

## Benefits

- Improves body flexibility and relieves muscle tension

- Stretches the spine and the back.

## 62. Drop back

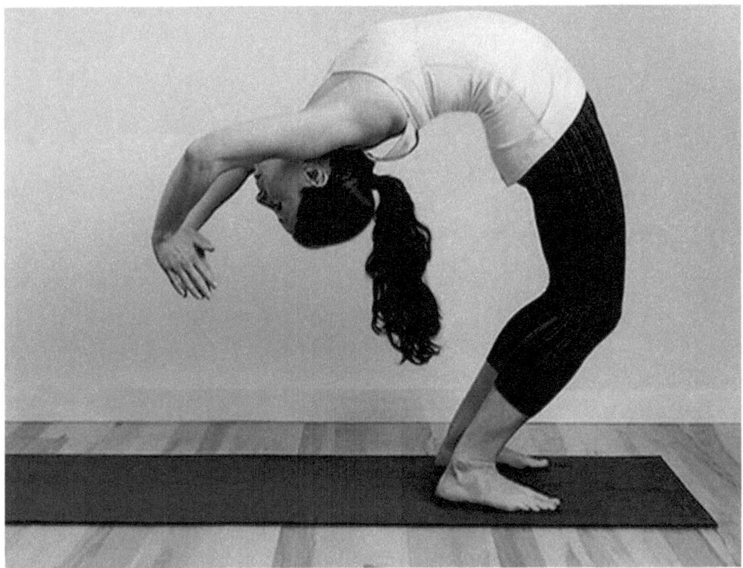

## Steps

- Begin by standing on your feet with your feet slightly apart

- Bend your knees as you stretch backward with the top of your head parallel to your butts or even lower.

- Stretch your arms forward then hold your palms together with your head between your arms

- Hold onto the position as you take 5 breaths.

## Benefits

- Stretches the back and spine muscles.

- Stretches the abdominal muscles

## 63. Standing Fly Crow

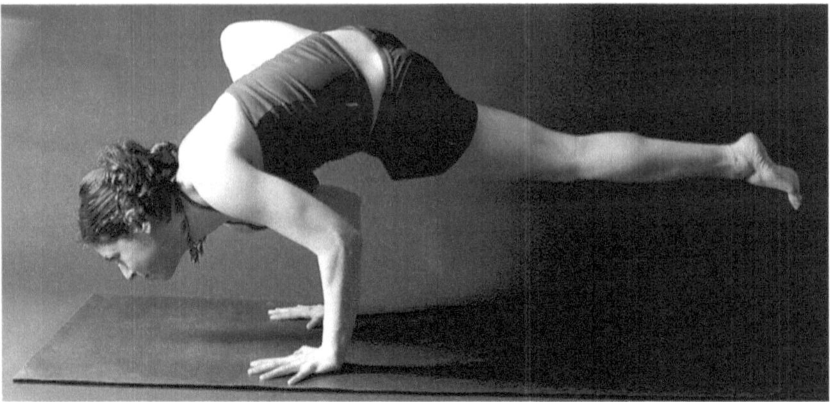

## Steps

- Begin by standing with your hips and feet a distance apart.

- Bend your knees as you sink the hips and reach out into chair pose

- Transfer the weight to the right foot then cross your ankle over to the right thigh as you flex your left foot and press on the left knee towards the ground.

- Place your palms on the ground with your shoulders a distance apart and in front of your rights shin.

- Stay in the position as you take five breaths.

## Benefits

- Strengthens the arms, wrists, neck, hips, and shoulders.

- Improves balance, focus and helps indigestion.

## 64. Locust Scorpion

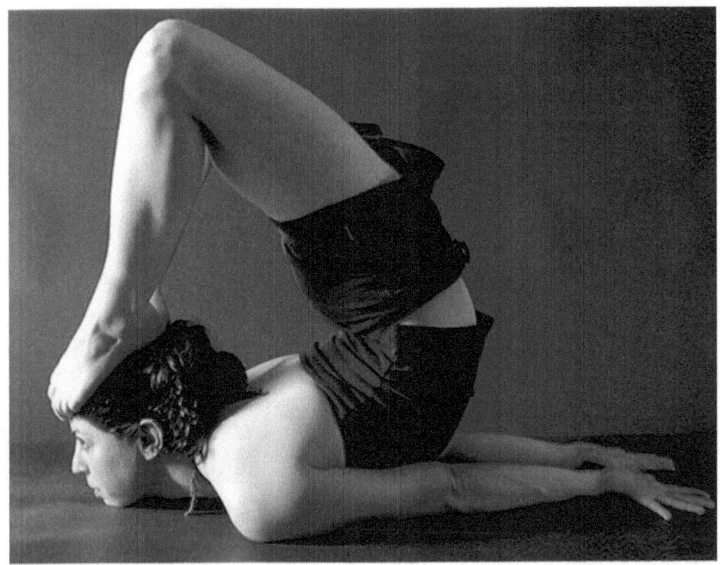

### Steps

- Start by lying on your belly and rolling over to your shoulders with your arms underneath you.

- Inhale as you press into the arms while lifting both the legs as high as possible.

- Bend your knees as you lower your feet and step on your head.

- Stay in the position for five deep breaths

### Benefits

- Strengthens the back and the spine and enhances flexibility.

- Stretches the entire body and improves blood circulation and digestion.

## 65. Lifted Thunderbolt

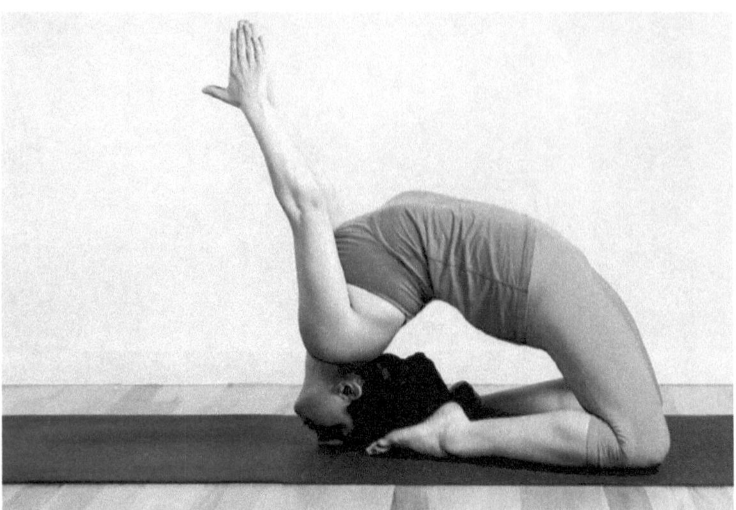

### Steps

- Begin with kneeling on the floor then bend backward until your head touches the floor right behind your bended knees as shown in the pose.

- Raise your hands straight with your palms open as if reaching out upwards.

- Stay in the position as you take five breaths

### Benefits

- Stretches the top of the feet and the body muscles.

- Increases blood flow to the head and the heart area.

## 66. Leg behind the head sage

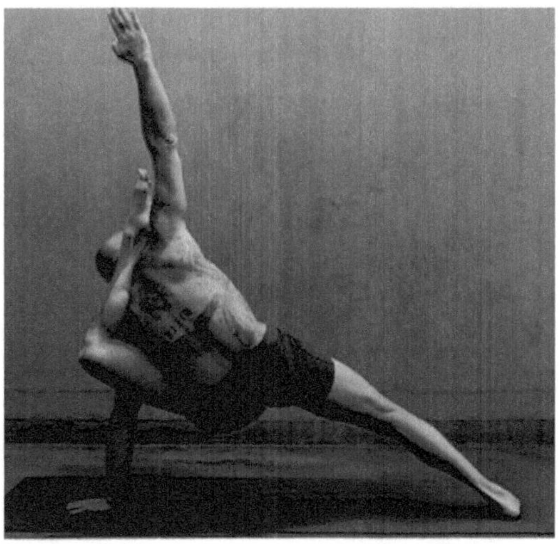

## Steps

- Begin with the downward dog position as you step your feet together

- Move your right hand to the left as you step your right foot forward then place your right foot on the floor with your toes pointing towards the left.

- Roll over to the right side then lift the left hand straight.

- Lift the left leg as you bend your knee and hold on to the big toe.

- Stay balanced in the position as you completely straighten your left leg.

- Keep your shoulders, hips, and spine straight.

- Release the hold on your left foot and place the left hand on the floor

- Stay in the position as you take five deep breaths while in the position

**Benefits**

- Enhances flexibility  of the hamstrings and the hips

- Improves body balance and strengthens the shoulder and upper body muscles.

## 67. Dancer Split

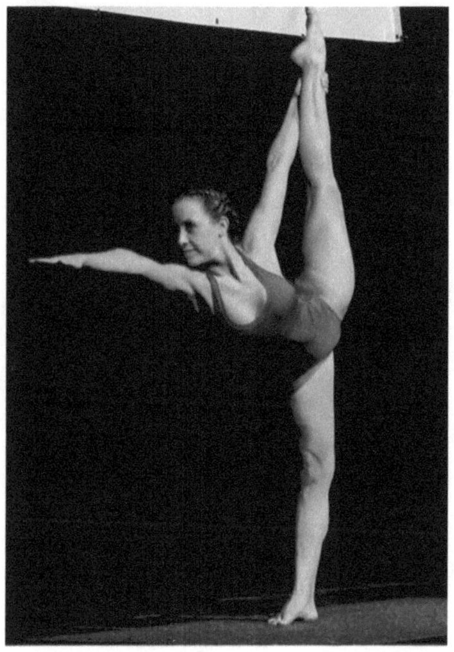

## Steps

- Start with mountain pose then inhale as your weight shifts to the left foot then bend your right knee.

- Reach out to the right foot with your right hand then grab your foot with the palms.

- Stretch your left arm in front of you as you focus your gaze in front of you in order to maintain balance.

- Stretch your right foot away as you lean the torso forward.

- Try and keep your chest open and the left leg straight

- Stay in the position as you take five breaths.

## Benefits

- Stretches the chest, shoulder as you increase flexibility in the spine and hips.

- Improves balance and blood circulation.

## 68.  Frog

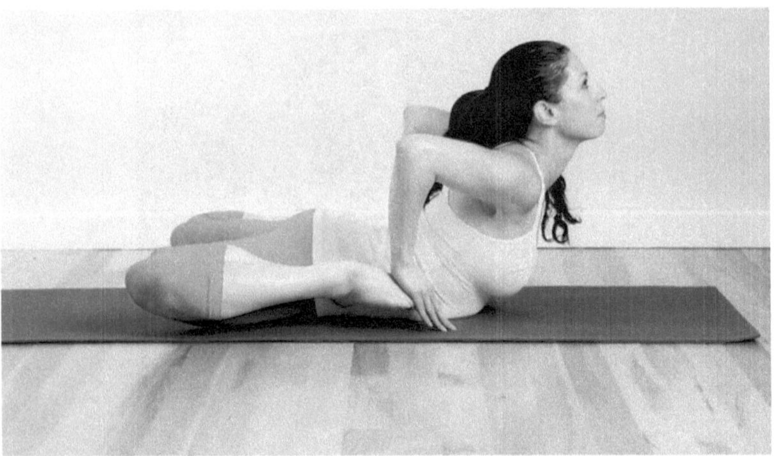

## Steps

- Lie on the floor with your belly as you prop the torso up with the elbows.

- Bend both of your knees as you reach the hands o grab your feet

- Turn your fingers to face the same direction like the toes then lift the elbows up to point towards the ceiling.

- Use strength from the upper body to press the soles of your feet towards the floor

- Lift the chest as high as possible then stay in the position as you take five breaths

## Benefits

- Stretches the thighs, shoulders and the chest

- Enhances flexibility of the muscles.

## 69. Pinching shoulders headstand

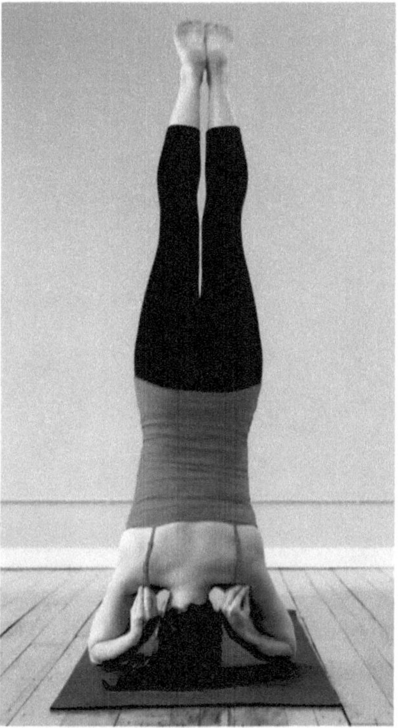

## Steps

- Begin by standing on your head with your feet stretched straight and together.

- Place your elbows on the floor and closer to your head with your fingers touching on your shoulders like in the pose.

- Take five deep breaths while in the position then relax and repeat again.

## Benefits

- Helps with activating the nervous system and awakens the mind.

- Increases breath rate and blood circulation

## 70. Yogic squat

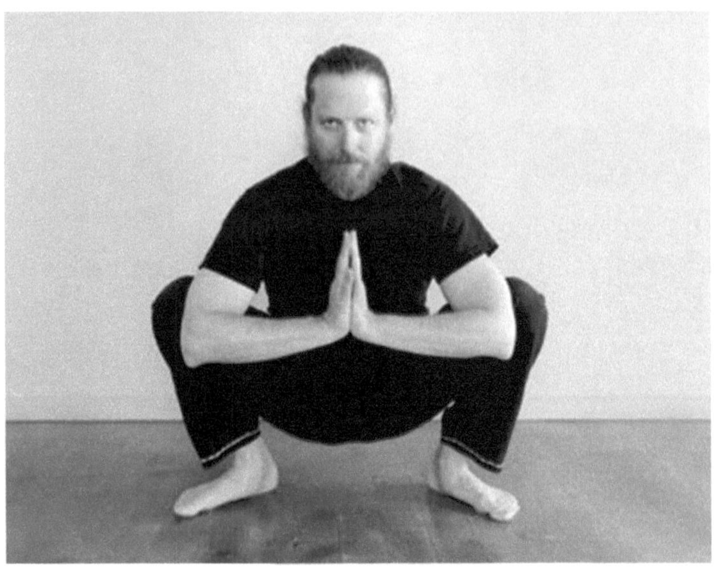

## Steps

- Place your feet shoulder distance apart then bend your knees so that your butt is at the lowest but don't hit the floor.

- Get your heels flat then squat straight with your hands in prayer pose and elbows pressing to the knees.

- Stay in the place for a few seconds as you breathe normally.

## Benefits

- Rehabilitates the flexibility in legs and the knees

- Relieves constipation.

## 71. Staff Pose

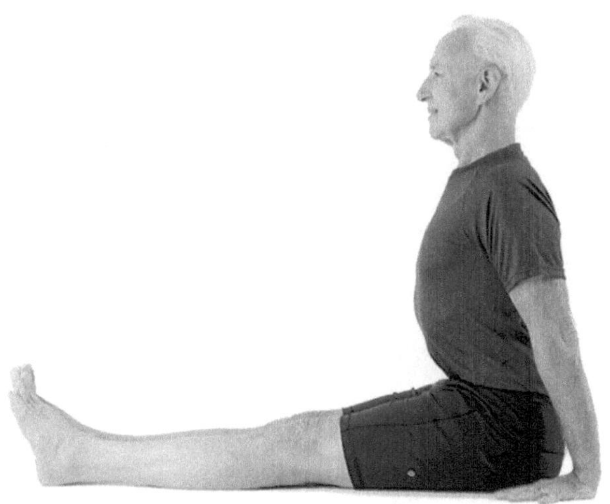

**Steps**

- Sit on the floor with your back straight and legs together straight.

- You can sit with your back against the wall for good alignment.

- The shoulder blades and your sacrum should touch the wall but not the lower back or back of your head.

- Place both your hands outside of your hips as in the pose above.

- Take deep breathes as you stay in the position.

**Benefits**

- Strengthens the back muscles

- Stretches the chest and the shoulders

- Improves body posture

## 72. Upward facing two-foot staff pose

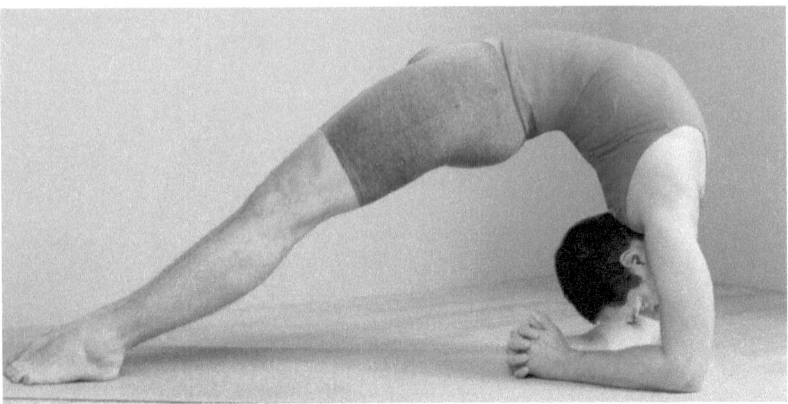

## Steps

- Lie on the floor on your back with your feet on the floor and heels beneath the knees.

- Straighten your feet wider than the hips then bend the arms as you place your palms on the floor near your ears, fingertips and your shoulders

- Pause as you focus on your breathing then exhale and press your knees against your torso.

- Lift your hips, shoulders and your head from the floor then straighten your arms.

- Bend your arms as you place the crown of your head as shown in the pose above

- Ensure that your legs are straight.

- Stay in the position as you take deep breaths.

## Benefits

- Stretches the body

- Opens up the chest and improves blood circulation.

## 73. Standing hand to big toe pose

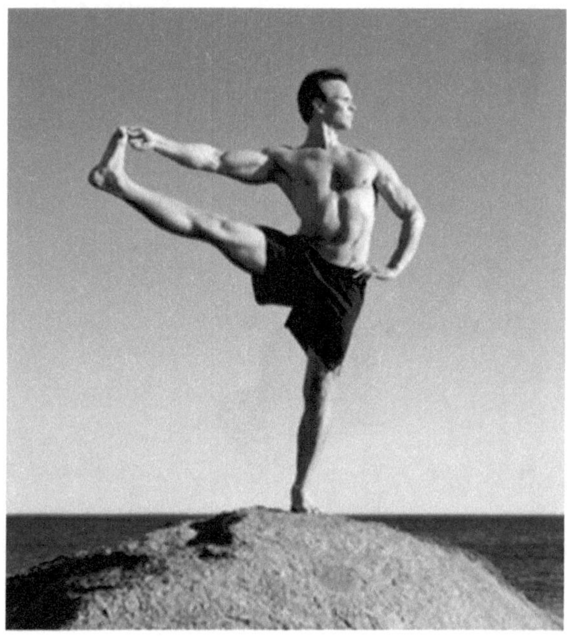

## Steps

- Stand by standing in the mountain pose with the feet together and arms by your sides.

- Shift that weight to the left foot then straighten your spine as you extend the right leg forward

- Ensure that your spine is straight and your shoulders relaxed.

- Hold onto the position as you take a few breaths then change to the right leg.

## Benefits

- Tones and strengthens he thighs, calves and ankles. It also stretches the hamstrings and opens up the shoulder blades.

- Enhances balance of the body ad stability

## 74. Lizard Lunge

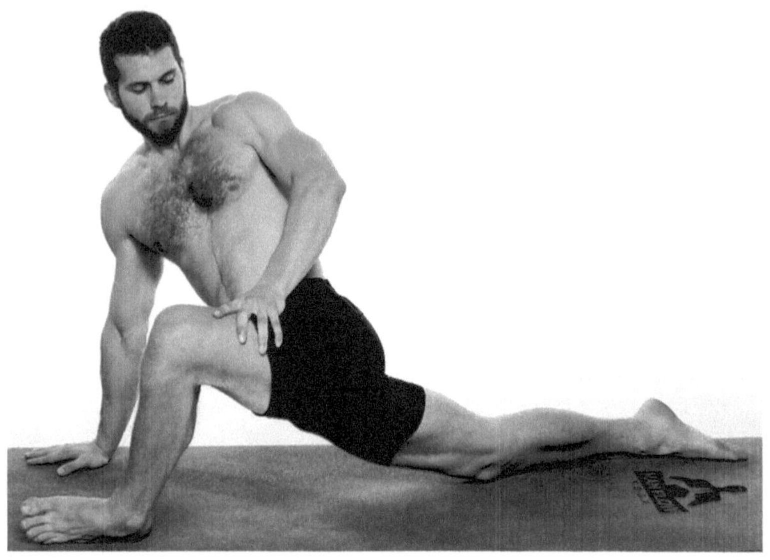

### Steps

- Bring the right foot outside the right hand as you come to the edge of your foot.

- Push your foot away from you slowly as in the pose then take 3 deep breaths.

- Twist to your right to intensify the pose then hold left ankle.

- Pull your foot close to the glutes as you bend your hip lower for a deeper quad and front hip stretch.

### Benefits

- Opens up the hip and targets muscles that are involved when running, jumping or squatting.

## 75. Crow pose

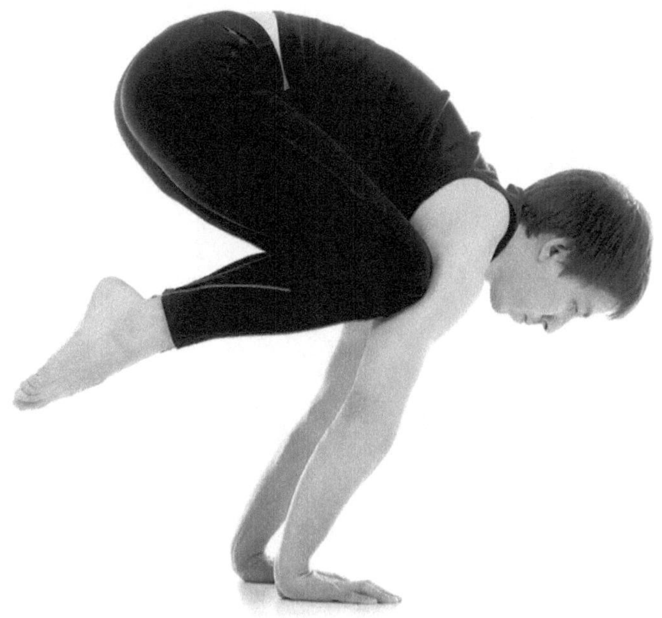

## Steps

- Place your hands on the floor then squat as you bring your knees to the armpits or even hug them close to your triceps.

- Engage your core and push forward as you distribute the weight to your hands with your knuckles grounded on the mat.

- Stay in the position as you monitor your breath.

## Benefits

- Balances the arm and enhances flexibility and strength.

- Improves blood circulation

## 76. Chair Pose

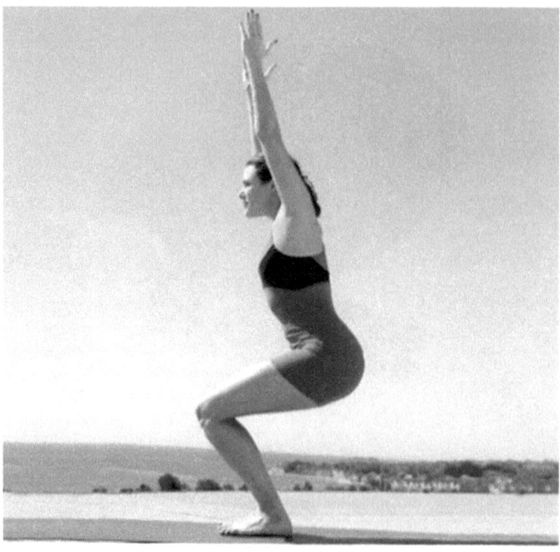

## Steps

- Start with the mountain pose with your touch closely touching

- Take a deep breath as you raise your arms over your head and perpendicular to the floor.

- Exhale as you bend the knees and bring your thighs parallel to the floor.

- Your knees should stretch outwards of your feet and torso as in the pose above.

- Draw the shoulder blades into upper back ribs and each your elbows towards your ears.

- Bring the hips down as you lift through your heart. Shift the weight to your heels

- Stay in the position as you keep your breath deep and smooth.

## Benefits

- Improves blood circulation and the metabolic systems.

- Stretches the shoulders while opening up the chest

- Tones the heart and the digestive organs.

## 77. **Reverse warrior pose**

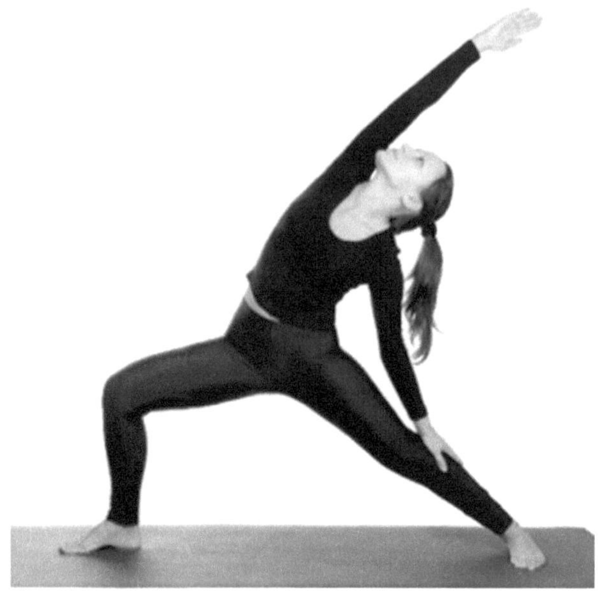

## Steps

- Start with the mountain pose as you stand with your feet and hips at a distance and your arms by the sides.

- Stretch the foot to 90 degrees as your toes point the top of the mat

- Raise your arms and your shoulder parallel to the floor

- Take a deep breath as you bend the front knee.

## Benefits

- Stretches and strengthens the groins, legs and hips, waist and the sides of your torso.

- Improves flexibility of the spine, ankles, inner thighs and the chest.

## 78. One legged head stand

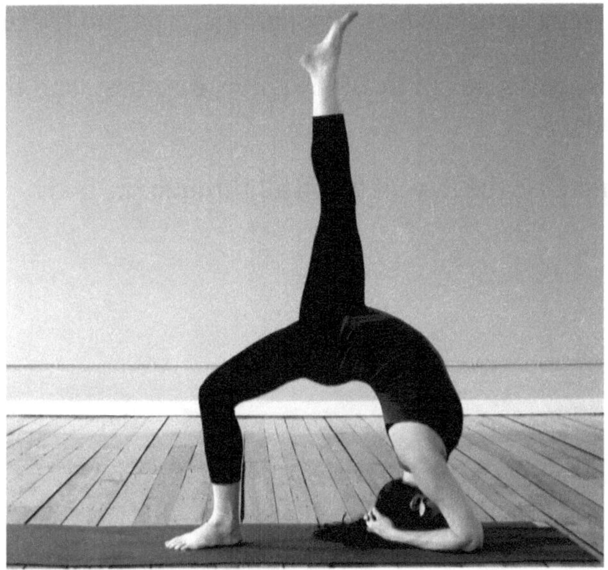

**Steps**

- Lie on the back then bend your knees as you place your feet on the ground with your wheel close to our bum.

- Bend the elbows as you place your palms on the ground above your shoulders with your fingertips facing your feet.

- Take a deep breath as you lift your shoulders and head into a wheel pose. Let the top of your head rest on the floor with your elbows bent and your fingers interlaced at the back of your head.

- Step both the feet forward as you step your left foot firmly on the ground.

- Raise the right leg into the air as you stay in the position for five deep breaths.

- Repeat the sequence again with the left sides.

## Benefits

- Strengthens the legs, hips, groins, hips and the torso.

- Improves flexibility of the spine, the chest, and the inner thighs.

- Increase the flow of blood all through the body.

## 79. Extended Locust Pose

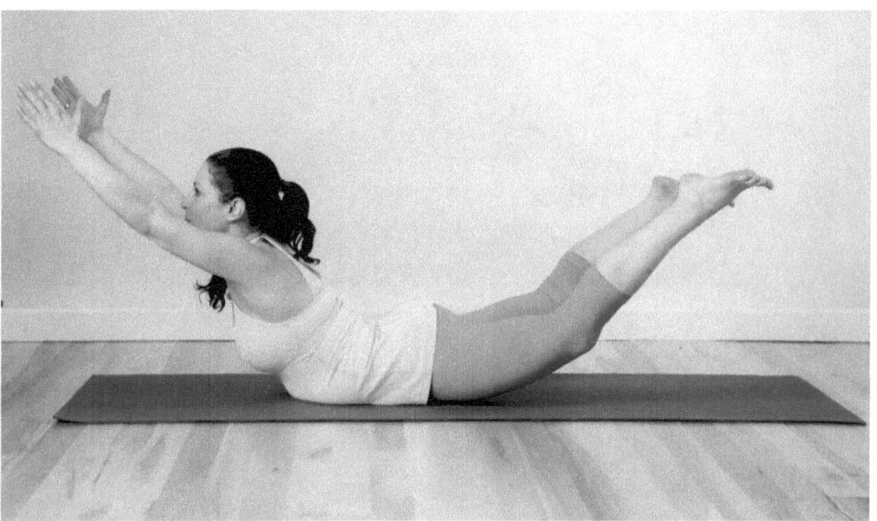

## Steps

- Lie with your belly on the floor as you stretch your arms straight in front.

- In hale as you lift your legs, the upper body and the head off the floor.

- Extend the crown of your head from your toes as you breathe while lengthening through your spine as you can.

- Keep the shoulders relaxed as you lift your arms and the legs as high as possible.

- Take five deep breaths then release back to your mat.

- Roll over as you come to a seated position with legs extended straight.

## Benefits

- Strengthens the entire back side and the body

- Improves the digestion system

## 80.    Burning lower lunge

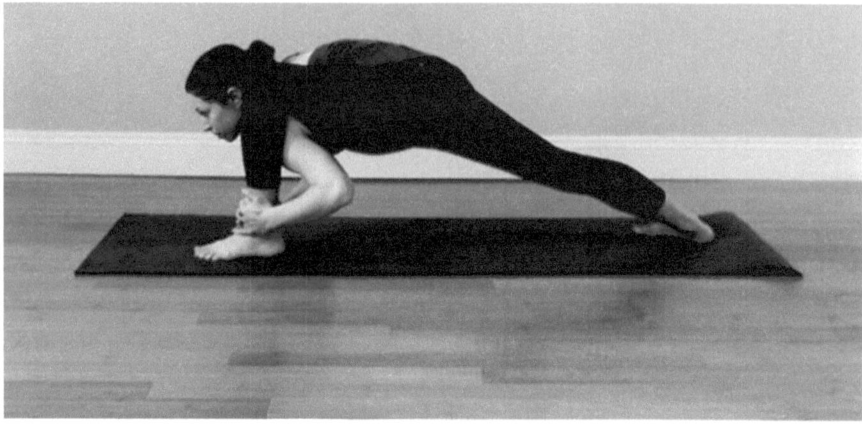

## Steps

- Lower your torso as you bend to reach your right arm under your bent knee

- Keep all the weight to your legs as you resist the urge of leaning into your hands

- Breathe deeply five times while in the position then step back.

- Repeat with the other side.

## Benefits

- Strengthens the lower parts of the body such as glutes, calves, and hamstrings.

- Tones the body

## 81. Extended Standing Straddle

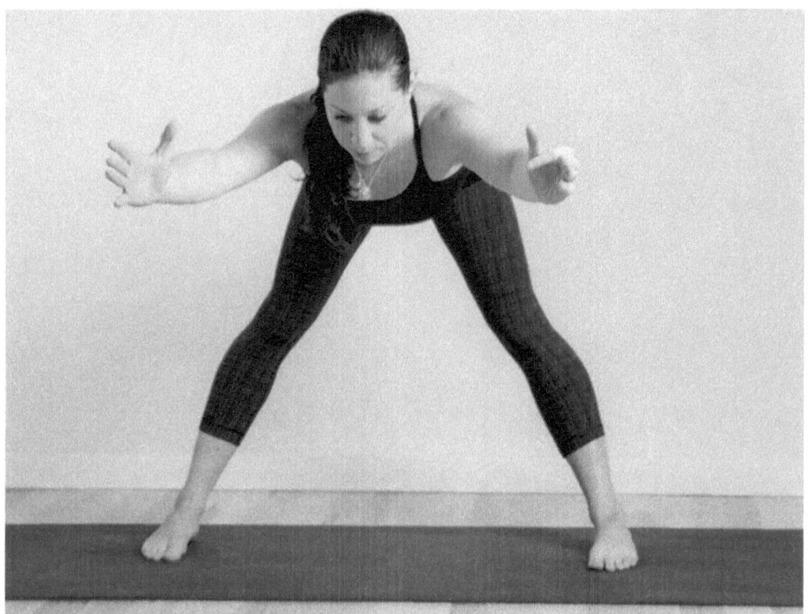

### Steps

- Stand in mountain pose with your left foot open as you face the left side of your mat.

- Inhale as you extend your arms straight in front of you.

- Exhale as you hinge at the hips, keep the back straight with your torso parallel to the floor.

- Draw your belly as you shift the weight towards your toes

- Stay in the place for about five breaths then step back to the mat.

### Benefits

- Strengthens your core, tush and the legs.

- Stretches the spine and the inner back legs.

## 82.Extended puppy pose

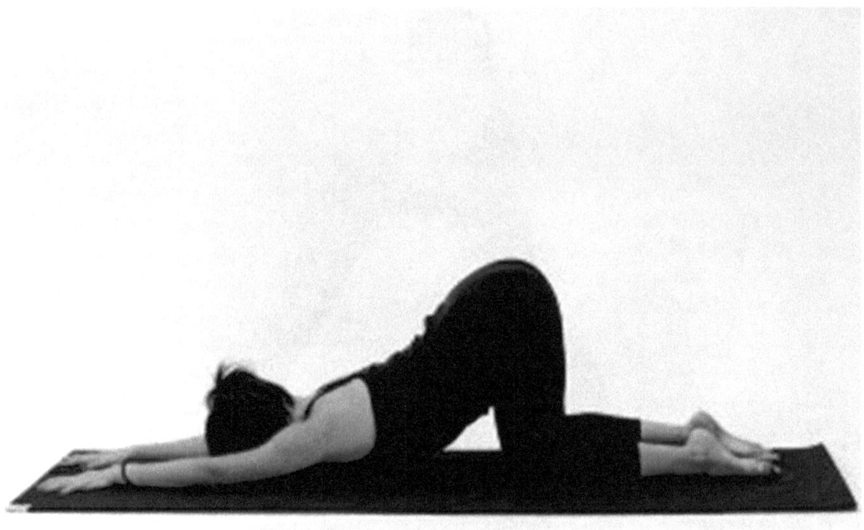

### Steps

- From the tabletop position lower your forearms then extend the arms long as you keep your hips over the knees.

- Move your hands forward as your arms stay engaged.

### Benefits

- Stretches the shoulders and the spine.

- Invigorates the body and calms the mind

- Strengthens the arms and stretches the hips and upper back.

## 83. Knees to chest

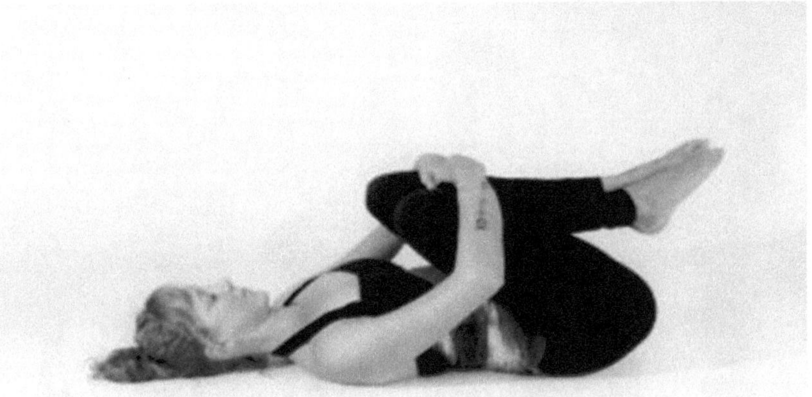

## Steps

- Begin by lying on the floor as you bring your knees to the chest and wrap the arms around the legs as if giving yourself a hug.

- Roll the shoulders away from the ears as you open your heart.

- Use your arms to squeeze and press the thighs towards the core then tuck your chin so as to elongate the top of your spin.

- Stay in the position as you as you take five deep breaths.

## Benefits

- Strengthens the biceps, triceps and other parts of the body.

- Lowers tension in the spine

## 84. Seated half spinal twist

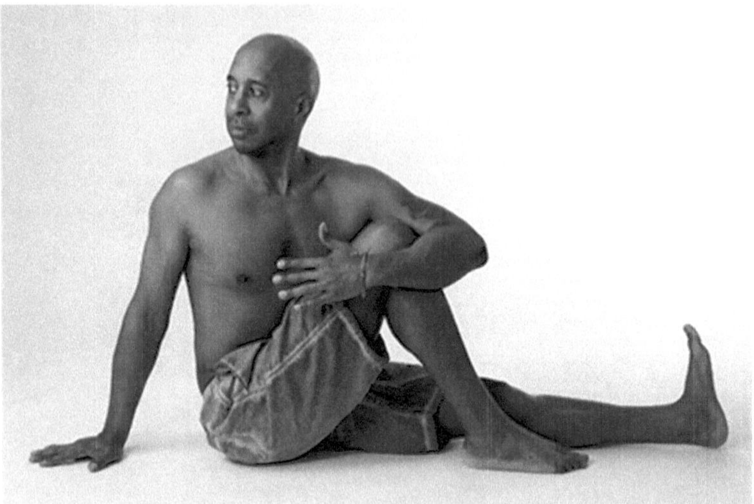

## Steps

- Sit down on the floor with your legs bent then drop your butt to the left of the legs

- Bend the right leg then cross then fold the right foot as shown in the pose

- Stretch your left arm and squeeze the right foot closer to your chest.

- Stay in the position as you take five deep breaths.

Benefits

- Strengthens and tones the abs

- Enhances flexibility of the hips and spine

- Expands shoulders and chest

- Relieves spinal and back pains.

## 85. Shoulder opener at wall

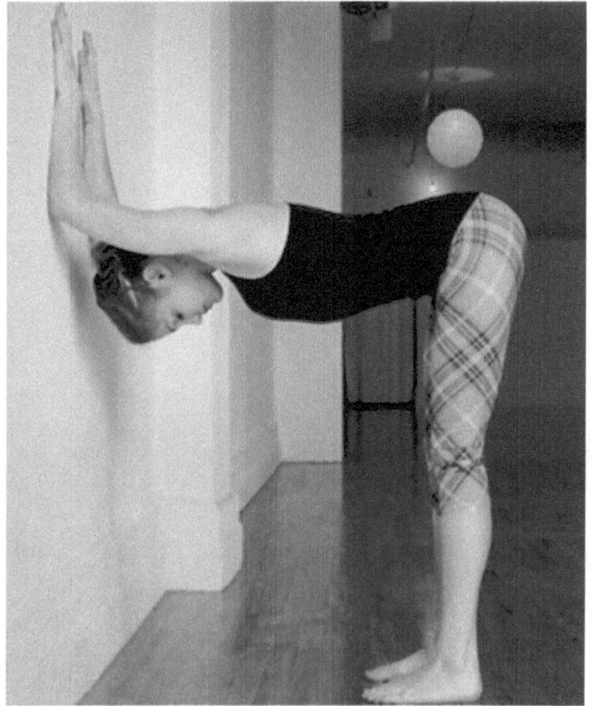

## Steps

- Place your arms on the wall below your shoulder height as you keep your elbows apart.

- Step back a few steps from the wall then allow your head to relax between your arms.

- Breathe while in the position for five deep breaths.

## Benefits

- Improves body posture and flexibility of the chest.

- Reduces stress and tension

## 86.  Crescent lunge with reverse prayer arm variation

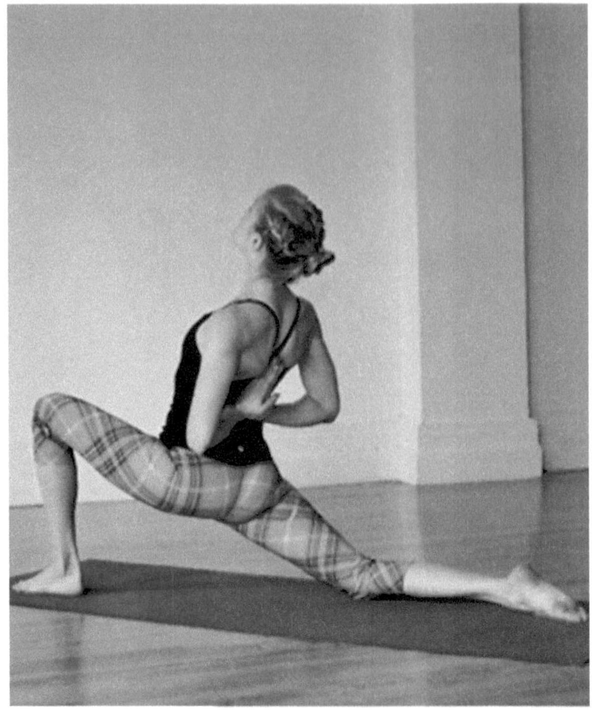

## Steps

- Take the down dog position then place the right foot forward as you place your left knee on the floor.

- Bend your elbows as you reach your arms behind the back and your palms pressed together in prayer position on your spine.

- Take five deep breaths while in the position then repeat with your right foot.

## Benefits

- Stretches the spine and back muscles

- Improves body flexibility and enlarges the thighs.

## 87. Forearm stand prep

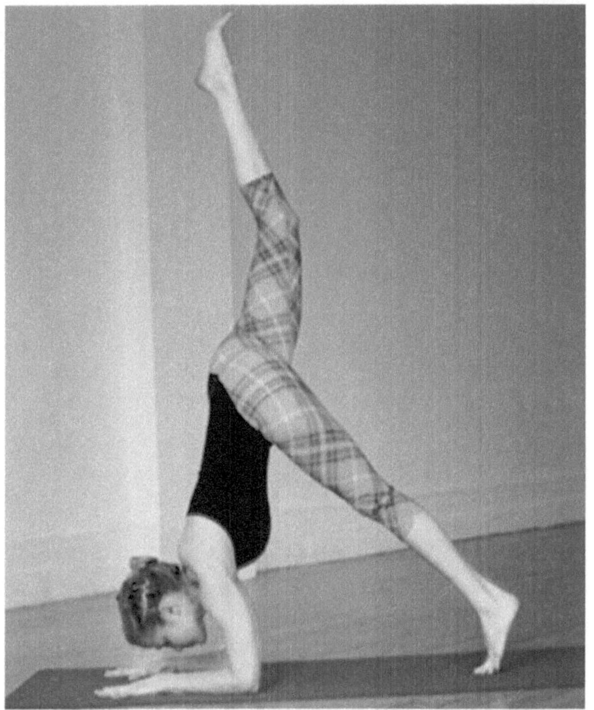

## Steps

- While in dolphin position, move your feet towards the elbows as you lift the right leg toward the ceiling.

- Take five deep breaths then repeat the pose with the left leg.

## Benefits

- Improves blood circulation to the brain and upper body parts.

- Enhances flexibility and stability

## 88. Hero's pose with cow face arm variation

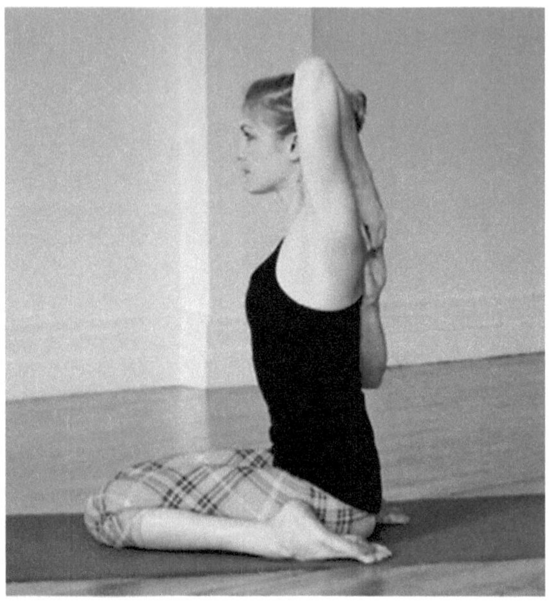

**Steps**

- Begin by kneeling on the floor then widen your heels until your thighs and feet are between your feet.

- Stretch the right arm towards the ceiling as you bend the right elbow and allow your hand to fall between the shoulder blades.

- Bend the left elbow as you reach your left hand towards your back and clasp the right hand.

- Take five deep breaths then release your arms as you repeat with the other side.

**Benefits**

- Stretches the hips, the knees, thighs, ankles, and feet

- Improves circulation of the blood and relieves flat feet

- Improves digestion and relief of gas.

## 89.  Reclining bound angle pose

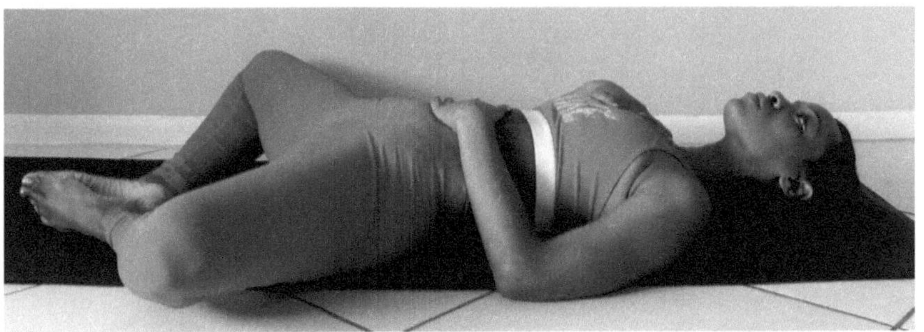

## Steps

- Lay on the floor with the legs extended and hands resting on your sides.

- Bend your knees towards the butt as you place the souls of your feet together.

- Let your thighs fall open gently towards the floor

- Res your hands on the floor or on the belly and at heart center.

- Take five long slow breaths while in the position.

## Benefits

- Great for enhancing sleep and stretches the hips and the thighs.

- Improves body posture

- Relieves tired legs

## 90.  Wall straddle split

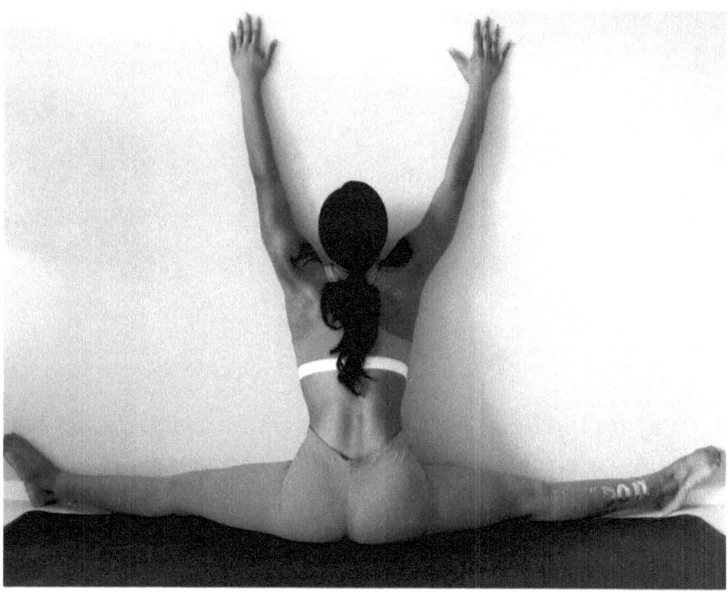

**Steps**

- Begin by sitting as you face a wall then open both your legs as shown in the pose.

- Press the chest towards the wall the shift your body as desired until you comfortably rest your hips and chest against the wall.

- Lift the hands high above the head then press your palms on the wall.

- Take five long and deep breaths while in the position.

**Benefits**

- Deeply stretches the thighs and opens up the hip flexors.

- Enhances body awareness and opens the hamstrings

- Improves perseverance

## 91. Revolved head to knee pose

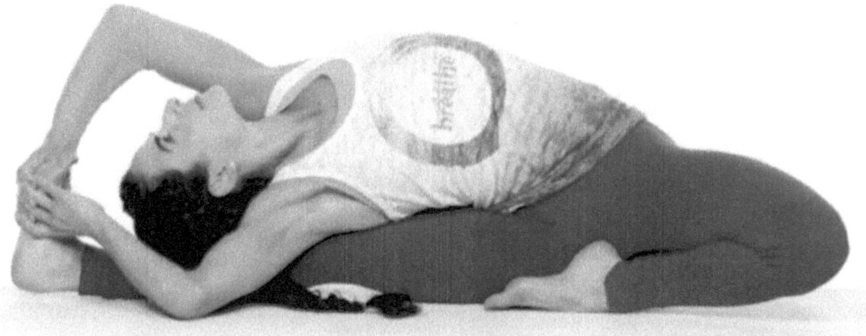

## Steps

- Sit on the floor with your legs wide and torso upright then bend your knee closer to your left groin

- Bend your right knee slightly as you slide the heel toward the right buttock.

- Lean towards the right as you press the back of your shoulder on your right knee. Place your right arm on the floor then lengthen our torso along the right thigh.

- Turn your palm toward the inner edge of the foot and your thumb on the top of your fingers, foot and the sole.

- Stay in the position as you take 5 deep breaths then change to the other side.

## Benefits

- Stretches the shoulders, spine, and hamstrings

- Stimulates abdominal organs like the kidneys, liver and improves digestion.

## 92. Cow face pose

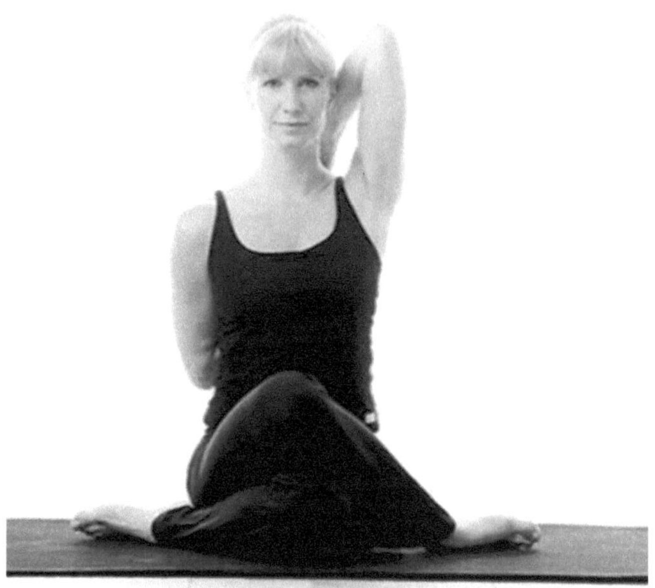

## Steps

- Sit in a staff pose then bend your knees and cross them as you place your feet on the floor

- Stretch your arms straight behind your back then hold them together as you inhale

- Stay in the position as you take 5 deep breaths then change your legs.

## Benefits

- Stretches the hips, ankles, and thighs.

- Exercises the triceps, the upper back of the body and chest muscles.

## 93.  Head to knee forward bend

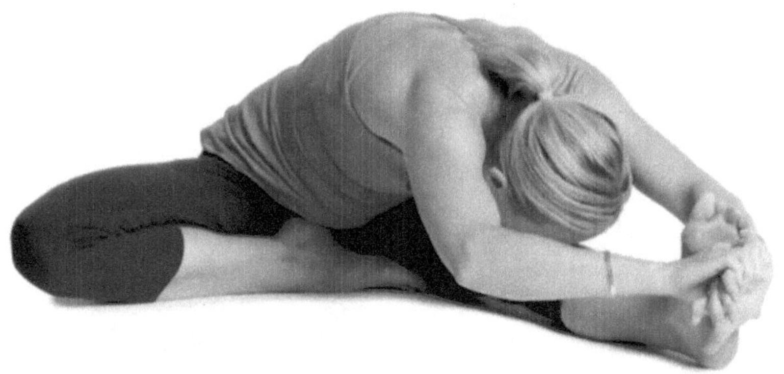

### Steps

- Sit on the edge of a firm blanket then stretch your legs in front of you as if in staff pose.

- Align your torso with the right leg then hold to the shin of your right leg.

- Let the belly touch your thighs and then the chest as your nose and the head touch your leg.

- Lengthen your torso with each breath and exhalation.

- Hold on to the breath for about 30 seconds then release and repeat 5 times.

### Benefits

- Calms the brain and helps with relieving mild depression

- Stretches the spine, hamstrings shoulders and the groins

- Stimulates the liver kidneys

- Improves digestion

## 94.Scale pose

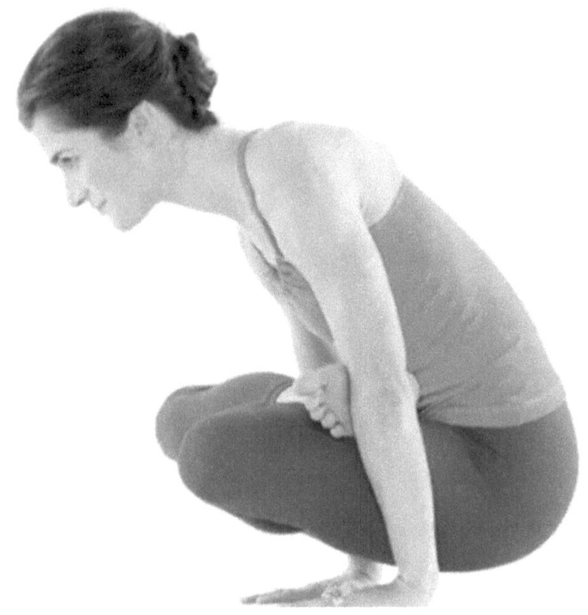

## Steps

- Place your palms on the floor beside the hips

- Take a deep breath as you push your hands on the floor.

- Lift your legs and butts from the floor as you contract the abdominal muscles.

- Hold onto the position for about 15 seconds then lower the legs and butts as you exhale.

## Benefits

- Strengthens the wrists, abdomen, and arms.

## 95. Sphinx pose

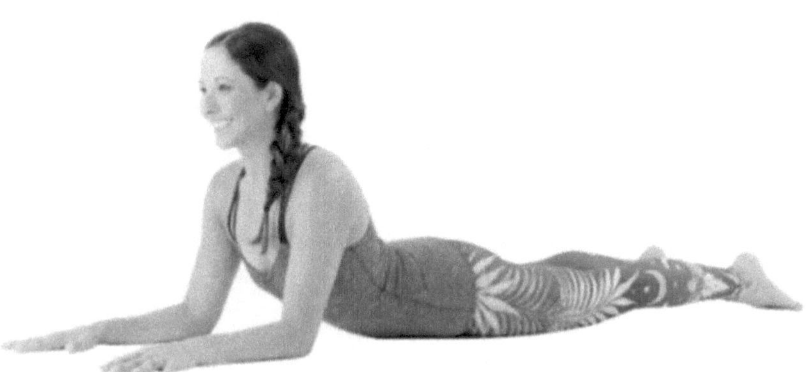

## Steps

- Lie on the floor with your belly on the floor and your feet stretched.

- Raise the upper part of your body and your head as your elbows and palms resting on the floor as shown in the pose.

- Stay in the position for 10 deep breaths.

## Benefits

- Strengthens the spine

- Stretches the chest, shoulders, abdomen, and lungs

- Firms the butts

- Stimulates abdominal organs and helps with stress relief.

## 96. Crouching eagle pose

### Steps

- Start by standing as you hug your right knee close to your chest then bend the left knee.

- Wrap the right leg around your left leg then wrap the right arm under the left arm as you press your palms together with the fingertips in the form of eagle pose.

- Sit down low as you keep your hips square and lift up through your fingertips and elbows

- Hinge forward at the waist then reach for the elbows in front of your knees.

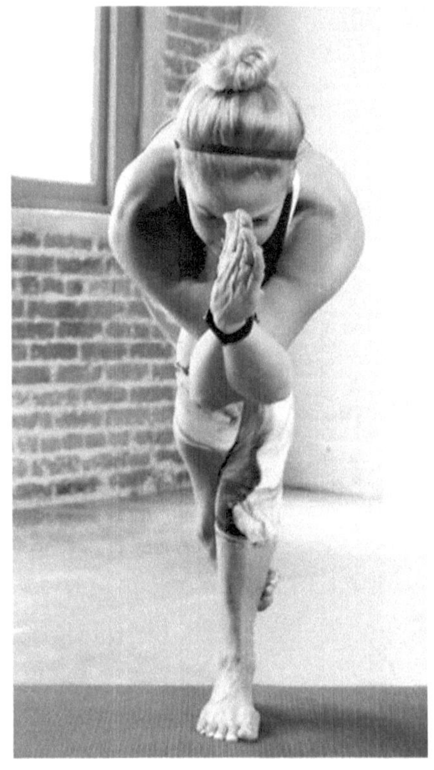

- The forearms should be parallel to the ground with the fingertips away from the face.

- Hold on to the pose for five breaths as you slowly unwind and repeat with the other side.

### Benefits

- Improves balance, focus, and concentration

- Enhances flexibility of the body.

## 97. Garland pose

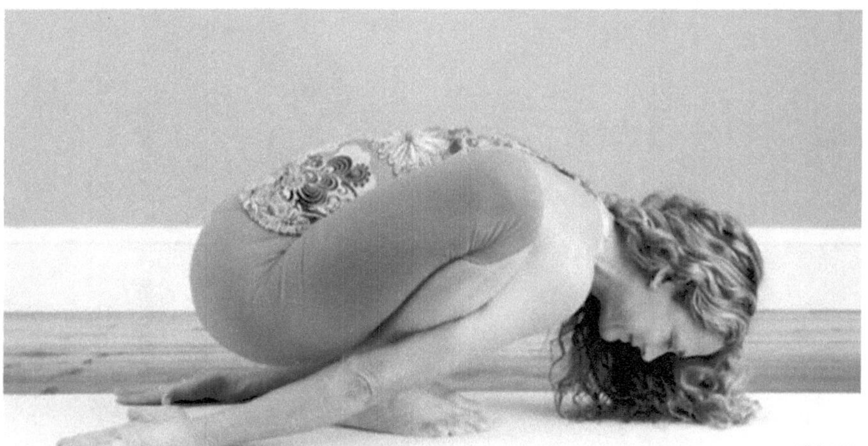

## Steps

- Place your feet together and knees wide with your torso in a forward fold.

- Wrap the arms behind your heals as in the pose

- Stay in the pose as you take deep breaths.

## Benefits

- Releases the lower back pains and opens the hips.

## 98.      Standing head to knee pose

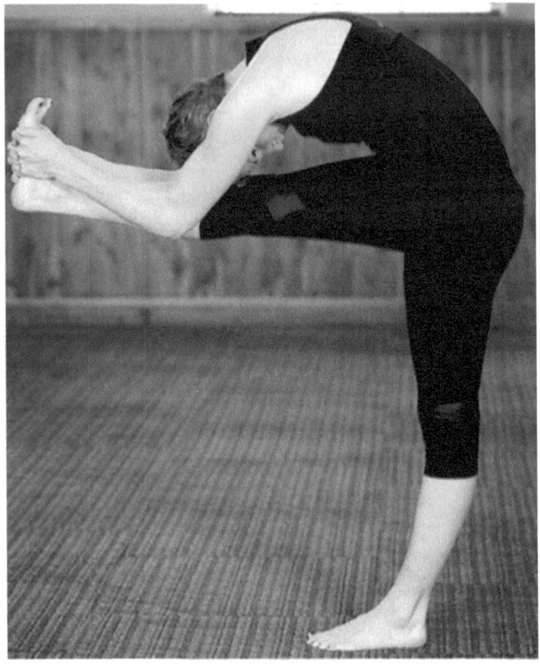

## Steps

- Stand on your feet with your legs apart then stretch your right leg and bend your head to rest on the raised feet.

- Stretch your arms and hold on to your foot with your hands clasped together.

- Stay in the position as you take 5 breaths or more.

## Benefits

- Builds mental strength while improving concentration

- Unifies the body and the mind and tightens thigh muscles and the abdominal muscles.

## 99.Marichi's pose

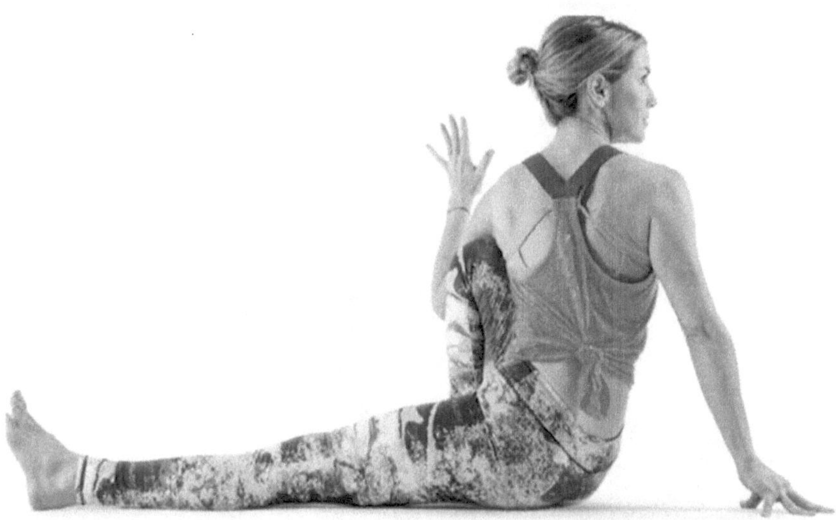

## Steps

- Sit in staff position as you bend your right knee and place your foot on the floor

- Put your heel close to the sitting bone as you keep your left leg strong while you rotate it slightly inward.

- Shift your shoulder with your head looking the opposite direction of your foot with one arm stretched up and another on the floor as per the pose above.

- Hold onto the position as you take 5 or deeper long breaths.

## Benefits

- Strengthens the thigh bones and tones the legs and arms.

- Stretches the hamstrings and the spine

- Enhances focus

## 100.        Peacock

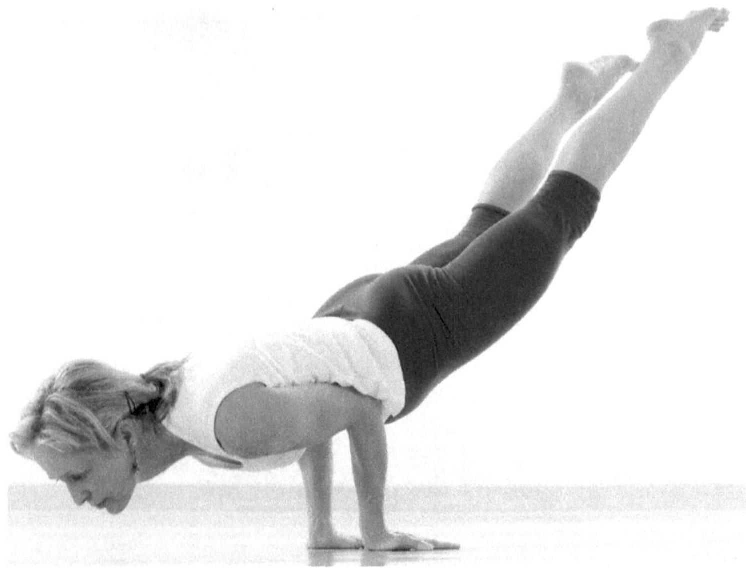

## Steps

- Kneel on the floor with your knees wide then bring your forearms and hands together and palm upwards.

- Lean forward as you place your hands flat on the floor and your fingers pointing towards the body.

- Keep the belly firm as your head drops towards the floor and your feet raised as in the pose

- Your body should be well aligned to the hands and in a parallel position to the floor.

- Stay in the position as you balance your breath.

- You can repeat it 3 times.

## Benefits

- Improves blood circulation and digestion

- Revitalizes the inner organs such as the pancreas, the liver, spleen and the stomach.

- Addresses constipation related cases and reduces acidity.

### 101.  Mountain Pose

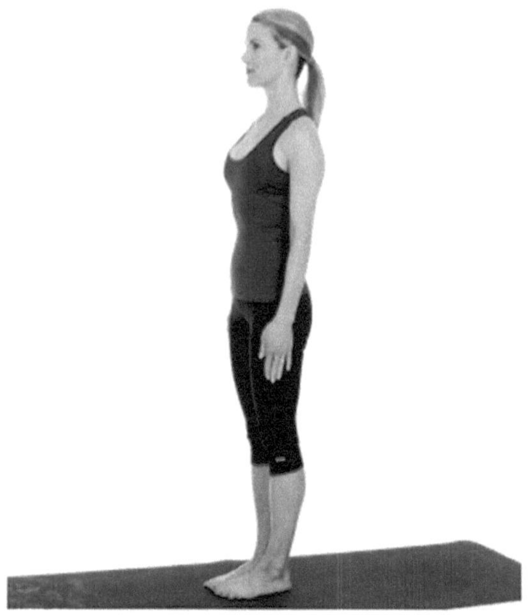

**Steps**

- Begin by standing straight with your feet closely together

- Lift your chest as you press the top of your shoulders down.

- Draw your abdomen in as you lift your chest

- Feel your shoulder blades come close to each other with the palms facing inwards towards the body.

- Take 5 - 8 deep long breaths while in the position.

## Benefits

- Improves body posture and strengthens the ankles, thighs, and knees.

- Steadies breathing and improves awareness.

- Firms the buttocks and the abdomen

**102.**        **Upward plank pose**

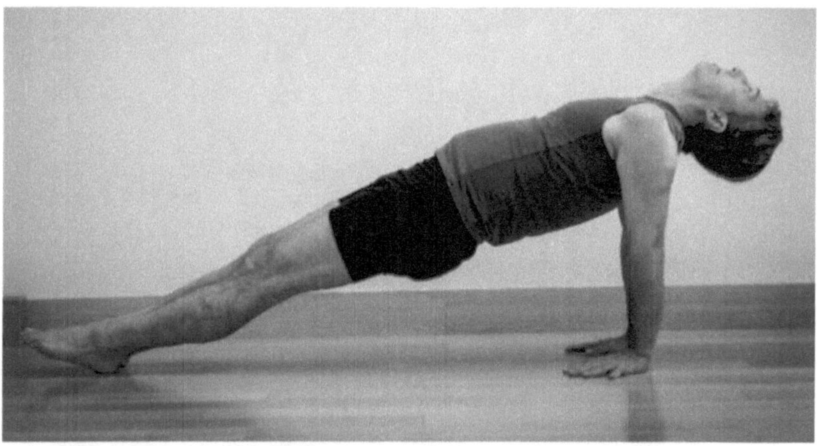

## Steps

- Start in a sitting position with your hands lowered behind your head and  pressing on the floor

- Stretch both your feet straight as you transfer the weight to your hands and lift your body off the floor.

- Stretch your legs as you place your heels on the ground with your toes raised.

- Stay in the position as you take five or more breaths

## Benefits

- Stretches and strengthens the shoulders, the arms, upper back, wrists, and glutes.

- Builds core strength while improving balance

## 103.    Formidable face pose

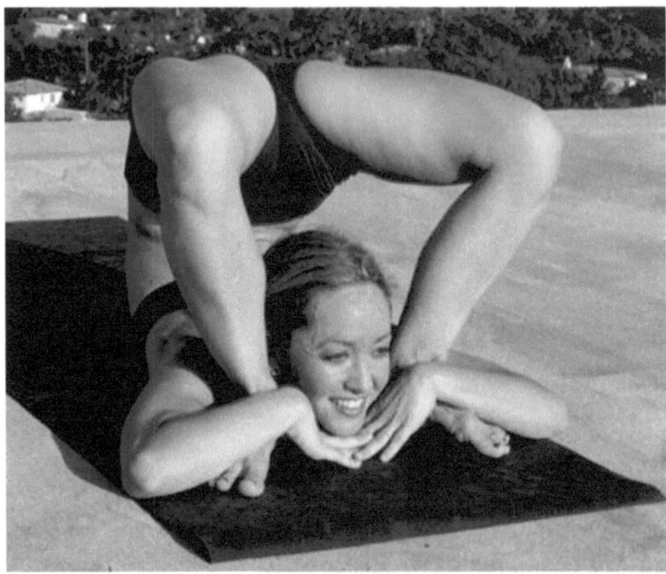

## Steps

- Begin with the downward facing dog pose then raise your right leg upwards

- Draw the right knee towards the nose and the right foot between your hands.

- Release the back knee to the floor then lift your chest and reach to the arms as you wrap your triceps forward as shown in the pose.

- Visualize your energy rise from the pubic bone to the navel

- Hold on to the position as you take five deep breaths or more.

## Benefits

- Stretches hip flexors and the quadriceps

- Opens up the chest, shoulders and back

- Lengthens the spine

**104.       Scorpion pose variation**

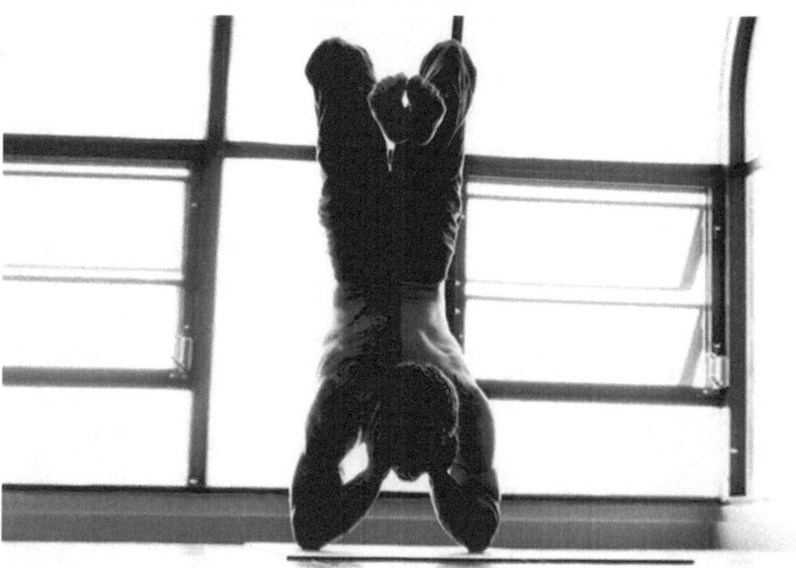

## Steps

- Start in the downward facing dog position then bring your forearms to the floor

- Place your elbows on the floor then raise your legs up as you transfer the weight to your bent arms.

- Bend your knees with your legs brought closer to the hips and feet stretched and held together.

- Raise your head and use your arms to support your head as in the pose above.

- Hold onto the pose as you take 5 or more deep breaths.

## Benefits

- Enhances optimal body strength and recovery from injuries.

- Strengthens the core, shoulders and overall body strength.

- Improves blood circulation

## 105.  One hand tree pose

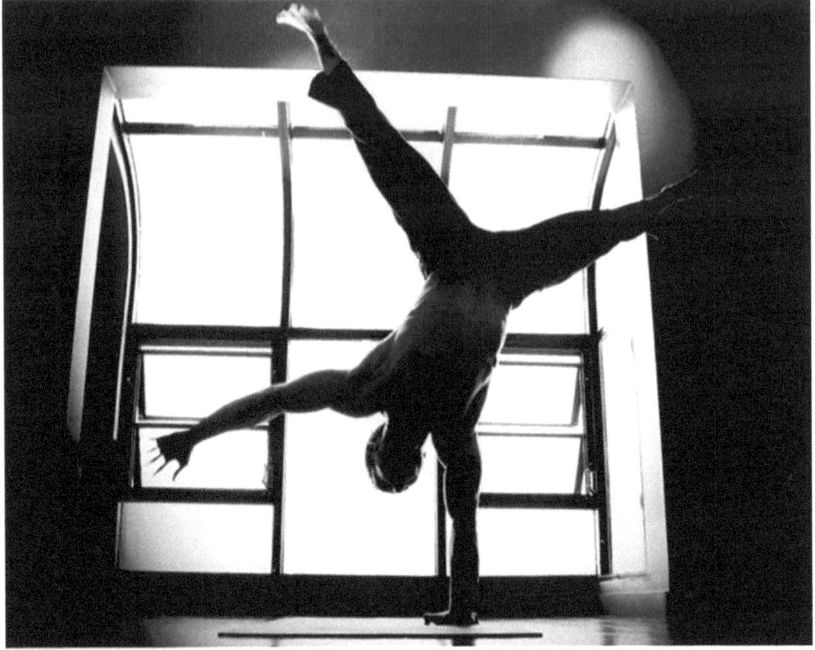

**Steps**

- Begin with both your hands on the floor and your legs upwards

- Release your left hand from the ground then stretch it as you transfer the weight to your right hand.

- Stretch your legs wide apart as shown in the pose above.

- Stay in the pose for 15 seconds as you adjust and gain balance then take 5 deep breaths while in the position.

**Benefits**

- Strengthens the leg, the ankles and foot muscles.

- Tones the arms and the shoulders

- Improves the ability to maintain balance and focus

## 106.  Tortoise Pose

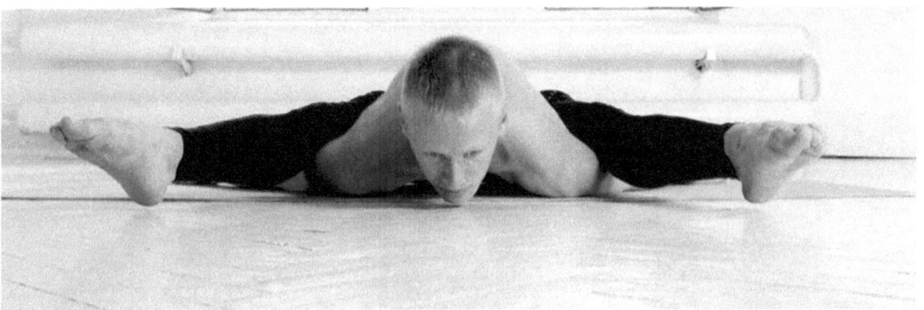

## Steps

- Sit with the legs straight in front of you and your hands also on the floor alongside your hips.

- Press your thighs on the floor as you lift your chest and flex your feet.

- Stretch your legs above your arms with your knees as wide as possible.

- Stay in the position as you take 5 or more deep breaths.

## Benefits

- Lengthens the spine and opens up the shoulders

- Quiets the mind as you prepare for meditation

## 107.   Horse pose

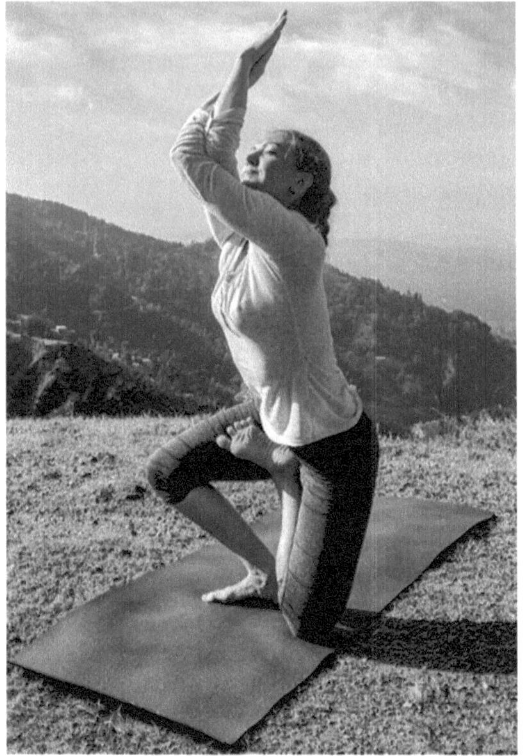

**Steps**

- Begin from a standing position then kneel on the left knee as you balance the weight between the two legs.

- Bend the right knee as you curve the left knee with the top of your foot resting on your right thigh.

- Bend slightly forward as you stretch your hands and cross them to overlap with both your hands together.

- Stay in the position as you take long breaths between 5 – 10 breaths.

**Benefits**

- Strengthens the muscles the legs and his inner thighs.

- Stretches the muscles

## 108.  Supine Spinal Twist

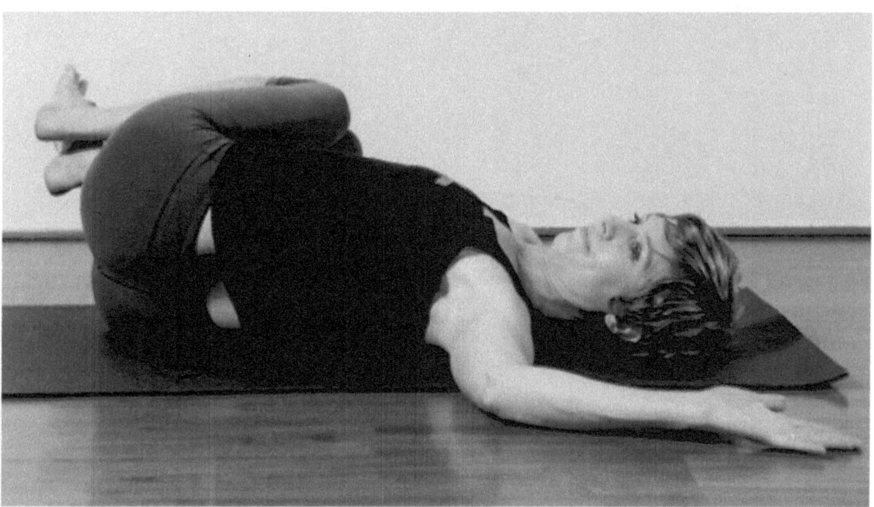

## Steps

- Begin with lying on your back then bring the arms out to your side and palms facing down

- Bend both the knees the twist your spine as you look towards the left fingertips

- Let the shoulders stay on the floor  then relax

- Stay in the position as you take five or more deep breaths.

## Benefits

- Stretches the back muscles, hydrates spinal discs, lengthens and realigns the spine

## 109. Supported Bridge Pose

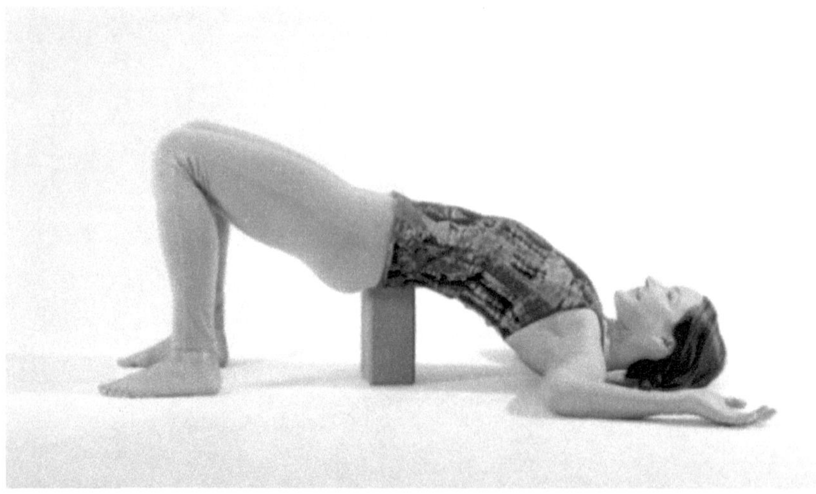

### Steps

- Begin with placing a block at a low medium level under the lower back

- Let your hips rest on the block as the shoulders stay on the floor with your arms wide apart outside your head.

- Stretch your thighs then res your feet on the floor as shown.

### Benefits

- Stretches the spine, neck and the chest.

- Stimulates the abdominal organs, thyroid, and lungs

- Improves digestion

- Relieves symptoms associated with menopause

## 110. Legs up the wall pose

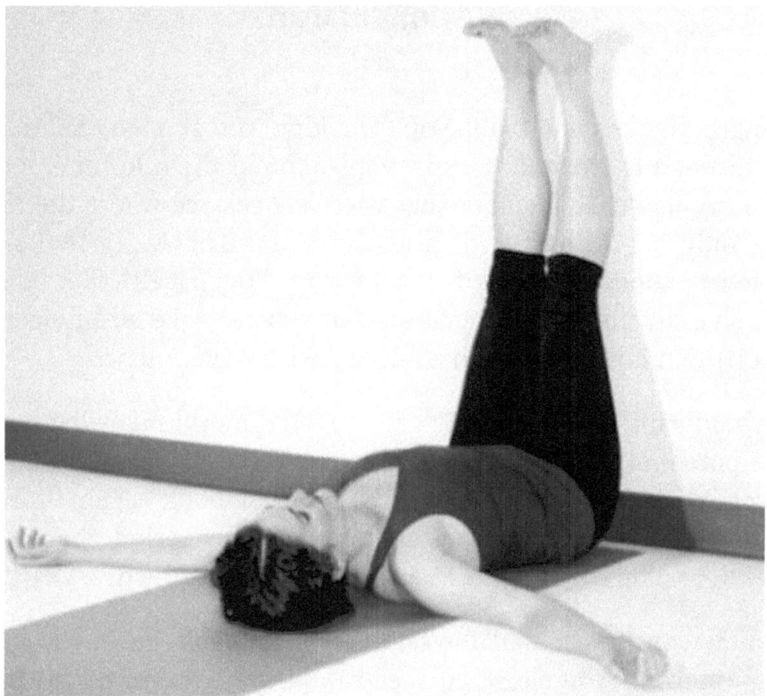

## Steps

- Place a folded blanket on the wall then lie down

- Stretch your feet up the wall as you keep the lower back elevated.

- Spread your hands straight as per the pose then take deep five breaths as you rest in the position.

## Benefits

- Relaxes the legs and entire body and great for those with insomnia.

- Improves blood circulation and breathing.

# Conclusion

Congratulations and thank you for taking your time to read this book all through to the end. I know you've found the information shared to be valuable. Remember that yoga is a science where the benefits can only be realized with practice. Yoga: The Best 110 Poses for Practice, Guide and Tips for Improving Your Health is a book that has shared valuable information that you can take advantage of and implement if you're to realize success with yoga practice.

He study and practice of yoga has revolutionized many lives and has the potential of impacting and improving every area of one's life. Take your time and go through the book again for solid understanding of the postures and the information shared if you intend to reap the benefits associated with yoga practice.

I know you have found the book to be valuable; however, I have a request would you please go ahead and leave a review for the book?

Thank you and enjoy yoga practice.